The Power of Us

The Power of Us

JAY VAN BAVEL & DOMINIC J. PACKER

WILDFIRE

First published in 2021 by
LITTLE, BROWN SPARK an imprint of LITTLE, BROWN AND COMPANY,
a division of HACHETTE BOOK GROUP, INC.

First published in the UK in 2021 by
WILDFIRE
an imprint of HEADLINE PUBLISHING GROUP

1

Cataloguing in Publication Data is available from the British Library

Hardback ISBN 978 1 4722 7414 4
Trade paperback ISBN 978 1 4722 7415 1

Offset in 11/16 pt ITC New Baskerville Std by Jouve (UK), Milton Keynes

Printed and bound in Great Britain by Clays Ltd, Elcograf S.p.A.

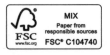

Headline's policy is to use papers that are natural, renewable and recyclable
products and made from wood grown in well-managed forests and other
controlled sources. The logging and manufacturing processes are expected
to conform to the environmental regulations of the country of origin.

HEADLINE PUBLISHING GROUP
an Hachette UK Company
Carmelite House
50 Victoria Embankment
London EC4Y 0DZ

www.headline.co.uk
www.hachette.co.uk

We are all a sort of chameleons, that still take a tincture from things near us.

—John Locke, *Some Thoughts Concerning Education*

Identity as area of interest, as the form in which you've chosen to expend your love—and your commitment.

—Zadie Smith, *Intimations*

CONTENTS

The Power of Us

INTRODUCTION

The room was abuzz with serious academic conversation. In the middle of it all stood the two of us trying to blend in by making small talk with a group of fellow graduate students. As new office mates, we hardly knew each other. Jay was a small-town kid from rural Alberta and Dominic a sophisticate born in England who'd relocated to Toronto from Montreal. Our relationship had encountered a rocky start a few weeks earlier when Jay adopted the spare old wooden desk in Dominic's office. Finding his tiny city apartment a bit cramped, Jay decided to bring his colossal and pungent bag of hockey equipment to store in our poorly ventilated sub-basement space.

The hockey bag had chilled our potential friendship, and at that point, we would have preferred to spend our time apart. But the opportunity for cheap wine and free food proved irresistible on our tight graduate-student budgets. For a few moments, we put aside our differences and debated the merits of using neuroscience techniques to study group dynamics. We were both genuinely excited about the possibility of using these new tools to look into people's minds as they interacted with others, formed teams, and struggled to confront their prejudices.

In a roomful of eminent scholars and hotshot young professors, we were at the bottom of the pecking order. But we didn't mind.

Every month, the University of Toronto's Department of Psychology hosted brilliant speakers from other universities, and we had the chance to take them out for lunch, grill them with questions at their talk, and join the entire department afterward for a catered gathering in the faculty lounge. To us, these were the most exciting events at the university, and for a few hours each month, we were invited to take part in these rituals.

But on this occasion, something went terribly, terribly wrong.

As we debated ideas, Jay popped a couple of pieces of cheddar into his mouth. The cheese had been cut into cubes roughly the size of dice. Someone made a witty remark. Jay, who was in mid-chew, laughed and then tried to swallow. Unsuccessfully, for at this moment, the cheese lodged firmly in his throat.

The conversation carried on. Nobody noticed Jay's sudden distress, the reddening of his face, the sheen of sweat forming on his brow. Not wanting to embarrass himself in a roomful of professors, he tried to wash the cheese down with a swig of beer. But instead of removing the obstacle, this made things worse, blocking any air from reaching his lungs.

Most people have experienced one or two terrifying life-and-death moments. Confronted with immediate danger, our brains set in motion a series of psychological and physiological responses that are designed to confront the threat. Our hearts start racing, our pupils dilate, and a rush of hormones are released to prepare for fight or flight. In those moments, the world seems to shrink as we focus on how to save our lives.

As if in slow motion, Jay saw Dominic and the other students turn to him with inquiring looks. Unable to speak, he clutched his throat in a choking motion. But it didn't register with the others. They looked on with confusion. A dozen jovial conversations continued in the background as if nothing were amiss.

Time was running out.

Jay scanned the room. He desperately wanted to impress the

faculty, and in the face of mortal peril, he felt caught between the need to save himself and an irrational desire to avoid public humiliation.

Suddenly an ancient memory from an old safety video came to mind, a lesson from one of the many safety courses he had taken while working in the oil fields of Alberta: people who are choking are more likely to die if they retreat to a private space like a restroom. If you stay in public and request help, usually someone will know how to administer the Heimlich maneuver to save your life.

Jay spotted the bartender a few feet away. One of the only nonacademics in the room, this man might have the training and presence of mind to save a student from choking on hors d'oeuvres. Jay stumbled behind the bar and, unable to speak, made another choking gesture. The bartender understood this universal sign of distress. He stood behind Jay, grabbed him around the midsection, and administered a few thrusts to the torso.

By now, professors and graduate students had noticed that something unusual was happening behind the bar. Conversations ebbed as people turned to stare at the two men wrapped in an awkward embrace.

The cheese was partially dislodged, and Jay felt a trace of air return to his lungs. Eager to avoid further embarrassment, he grabbed Dominic by the arm and pulled him through the crowd and out of the reception. There was a men's room across the hall and Jay, still struggling to breathe, needed more help.

It was then that Dominic fully understood the situation. It had been years since he'd learned the Heimlich maneuver at summer camp and he wasn't sure that he remembered what to do. But realizing that he was all that stood between Jay's future as a psychologist and his imminent demise in the restroom, Dominic wrapped his arms around his new office mate.

After a few hesitant pumps, Dom got the hang of it, and with one final push of his fists into Jay's midriff, the cheese popped out and rolled across the floor!

Jay took a long, deep, thankful breath of relief.

We stared at each other.

Our immediate reactions to this near-death experience could hardly have been more different. As professors came in and out of the men's room giving us strange looks, Jay laughed uproariously at the absurdity of the situation. The thought of dying at a wine-and-cheese seemed too surreal to be taken seriously. He wanted to head back to the reception for another round of drinks and some more cheese before the platter was bare.

Dominic, however, was aghast, shaken by the gravity of what had just occurred. The last thing he wanted to do was watch Jay attempt to eat more cheese.

But the stress of the situation was mutual and had a deeper effect. It was this upsetting—and somewhat humiliating—event that started the two of us on a path toward becoming a scientific team. We were no longer just two individuals tolerating each other in our small sub-basement office but a pair of resilient young scientists bound together by a shared brush with death at a colloquium event.

In the weeks that followed, we began turning to each other more and more often to talk about research. The odorous bag of hockey gear no longer stood between us (though Dom was quietly relieved when Jay eventually moved to a bigger apartment and took it away). Before long, we were developing shared ideas, designing experiments, and analyzing data together. Our other office mates surely found our endless banter tiresome, but we were happy in our windowless existence.

Our harrowing choking incident was the beginning of a bond that would strengthen throughout graduate school and persist as we both became postdocs at The Ohio State University and later became professors ourselves at universities on the East Coast of the United States. Together, we joined the community of social psychologists and, more generally, of scientists. Later, within a few weeks of each other, we joined the wonderful and exhausting world of parenting. And now, together, we have become authors. All of these things are central parts of our identities.

As social psychologists, we study how the groups that people belong to become part of their sense of self—and how those identities fundamentally shape how they understand the world, what they feel and believe, and how they make decisions. That's what this book is about.

Together with you, we will explore the dynamics of shared identities. What causes people to develop a social identity? What happens to people when they define themselves in terms of group memberships? And how can shared identities improve performance, increase cooperation, and promote social harmony—as they did in our own office?

In this book, we will explore the power embedded in this feeling of "us." We will explain how the dynamics of identity are key to understanding a great deal of human life. The philosopher Aristotle famously said that "knowing yourself is the beginning of all wisdom." But we will argue that truly knowing yourself is not about trying to pin down an essence, a stable and immutable command of who you are. Instead, knowing yourself is about understanding how your identity is shaped and reshaped by the social world that you are inextricably embedded in—as well as how you shape the identities of people around you.

Understanding how identity works provides a special type of wisdom: the ability to see, make sense of, and (sometimes) resist the social forces that influence you. It also gives you the tools to influence the groups you belong to. Among other things, you can learn how to provide effective leadership, avoid groupthink, promote cooperation, and fight discrimination.

We aim to provide a deeper understanding of identity, an understanding that allows people to move beyond inquiring "Who am I?" to asking "Who do I want to be?"

CHAPTER 1

THE POWER OF US

Herzogenaurach is an idyllic town in southern Germany named for the river Aurach that flows through it. The river serves as a dividing line between two fierce rivals.

The saga began, as many do, with two brothers. The Dassler brothers—Adolf (Adi) and Rudolf (Rudi)—were cobblers, and before the Second World War, they made shoes together. From humble beginnings in their mother's laundry room, they founded the Gebrüder Dassler Schuhfabrik and specialized in producing athletic footwear.

The brothers' factory made the shoes that Jesse Owens, the Black American track star, wore for the 1936 Olympics in Berlin; Owens was wearing these shoes when, much to the chagrin of the German führer, Adolf Hitler, he won four gold medals. His victory gave the brothers international exposure, and sales of their shoes exploded.

No one is sure exactly how the brothers' conflict started. But according to legend, the rivalry was triggered by a bombing raid in 1943. Adi and his wife climbed into the same shelter as Rudi's family, and Adi exclaimed, "The dirty bastards are back again." Although Adi was probably referring to the Allied warplanes, Rudi apparently believed the insult was intended for himself and his family.

After the war, Adi and Rudi began a battle that would inflame and divide their hometown for decades. The Dassler brothers' shoe company did not survive. By 1948, the brothers had split the business, and Herzogenaurach became home to two of the largest shoe manufacturers in the world. On each side of the river, brand loyalty dominated.

These two shoemaking behemoths, collectively worth more than twenty-five billion dollars today, became bitter crosstown rivals. The conflict spread to employees and their families. The town's citizens identified exclusively with Adi's or Rudi's company. Walking about town, people would look down at each other's shoes, making sure that they interacted only with members of their own group. Thus did Herzogenaurach become known as the "Town of Bent Necks."

In her book *Pitch Invasion*, Barbara Smit describes how each side of the town had its own bakeries, restaurants, and stores.[1] Townsfolk from the other side were refused service if they wandered into the wrong establishments. Families were divided. Once-friendly neighbors became enemies. Dating or marrying across company lines was also discouraged! It wasn't until the Dassler brothers died that the tensions eased and the companies established a rivalry that today is focused more squarely on business and the soccer pitch. But the brothers took their enmity quite literally to the grave: they are buried at opposite ends of the town's cemetery.[2]

The companies they formed live on. You know them as Adidas, founded by Adi, and Puma, founded by Rudi. The mayor of Herzogenaurach recently explained, "I was a member of the Puma family because of my aunt. I was one of the children who wore all Puma clothes. It was a joke in our youth: you wear Adidas, I have Puma. I'm a member of the Puma family." It wasn't until 2009, after Adi's and Rudi's deaths and decades of hostility, that the employees from both companies marked an end to the feud by playing a friendly soccer match.

The striking thing about the long and hard-fought battle initiated by the Dassler brothers was that it didn't stem from something one might consider weighty or important enough to divide a town. It wasn't about politics or religion. It wasn't about land, gold, or ideology. It was about shoes. Or, more accurately, it was about opposing identities based on shoes. Once these social identities were created, they exerted tremendous power, dictating where employees, their families, and subsequent generations lived, ate, and shopped.

The critical question, however, is not why the Dassler brothers went to war over shoes. After all, brothers have been among the most jealous of rivals since Cain and Abel. The question is why everyone else went along with it. Why did the rest of the town so readily embrace one side over the other?

PSYCHOLOGISTS ON A PLANE

When we travel, after squeezing our luggage and ourselves into cramped airline seats, we often end up in conversation with friendly strangers. These chats tend to follow a familiar rhythm. "Where are you from?" "Why are you going to Dallas [or Portland or Sydney or Taipei]?" And, of course, "What do you do?"

"Oh, um, I'm a psychologist."

Nine times out of ten, this elicits the same reaction. "Uh-oh—are you analyzing me? Can you read my mind?"

We usually laugh and brush it off. "Ha-ha, don't worry—I'm not *that* kind of psychologist." Every once in a while, though, just for fun, we give it a shot.

We are social psychologists and, even more specifically, psychologists who study social identities. We study how the groups that people identify with affect their sense of self, how they perceive and understand the world, and how they make decisions.

If they wanted to analyze a fellow passenger, other types of psychologists would ask different questions than we would. A clinical

11

psychologist might ask you about feelings of anxiety and depression or about family histories of mental illness. An old-school clinician might ask you about your dreams or your relationship with your mother. Personality psychologists might whip out a Big Five trait inventory and measure your levels of extraversion, conscientiousness, and openness to experience. Others could inquire as to your birth order or the experiences in your life that you believe were most formative.

We would ask you about your groups: *What groups are you proud to belong to? What group memberships do you find yourself thinking about a lot? Which ones affect how you get treated by other people? With which groups do you feel solidarity?*

The answers to these questions give us some useful clues about who you are. We assume that you will tend to conform to the norms of these groups, enjoy their traditions, and feel pride in their symbols. We also expect that when you dissent and really speak your mind, it will be in these groups. This might seem surprising, but dissent is quite hard and people are often willing to do it only because they care deeply about a group.

We can infer that you will tend to like and trust fellow members of these groups and that you might be willing to sacrifice your own resources or well-being, if necessary, on their behalf. If any of your groups have serious rivals, we can also predict how you feel toward members of those groups and how you might treat them. And if we learn that you think one of your important groups is being treated unjustly, we have a pretty good sense of how you might vote, the causes you're likely to join, and who you will fight for.

There is, of course, much more to you than that. But this is just about as much analysis as anyone wants while stuck next to a stranger thirty thousand feet in the air!

When people travel and have these sorts of conversations, they often form a small, fleeting bond with each other. But these rarely turn into anything more. They rarely become part of someone's identity, for example.

In this book, we will talk a lot about how groups actually do become parts of our identities, so we should clarify what we mean by these terms. Fifty or one hundred and fifty people together on a plane are not a group—at least, not psychologically. They are simply a collection of people who, for the moment, share the same cramped space, stale air, and unappetizing food choices. But they lack a sense of solidarity, of being a collective, of sharing a bond. They do not possess a meaningful social identity as passengers.

Most flights pass entirely in this fashion. The flight attendants are probably a group and share a sense of identity, as are families or coworkers traveling together. But the plane's passengers, as a whole, are not.

Circumstances can change this, giving rise to a feeling of collective solidarity, even if only momentarily. On a stormy night a couple of years ago, Dom was flying home along the East Coast of the United States. From their tiny windows, the passengers could see a line of thunderstorms—massive dark towers of clouds, lit up eerily every few seconds as lightning coursed through them. As the plane flew north, the pilots weaved their way between the clouds. It got rough, the small commuter plane jerking and shaking, creaking ominously. "We're hitting a bit of turbulence, folks," one pilot announced over the inevitably scratchy intercom, "but don't worry, we think we're gonna be okay!"

The words *we think we're gonna be okay* did not have the intended effect. Now people began to look at one another with unease. Conversations started between rows. Over the churning sound of the engines, passengers recounted stormy flights they'd had in the past, assuring one another that it would indeed be okay. And it was. The plane eventually escaped the storms and landed just fine, even on time.

But the psychology of that flight was different than normal. The common experience that everyone had been through was a foundation for a momentary collective bond and a sense of community. The passengers had survived something stressful and unique together. When the plane landed, everybody applauded. For a while together, they had shared an identity.

In this chapter, we will lay out some of the principles of identity that will provide a foundation for the rest of the book. This is one of them: although we have enduring, strong, and deeply meaningful long-term social identities, human psychology also provides us with a readiness to connect with each other in momentary solidarity. Some situations, such as administering the Heimlich maneuver to a colleague or hoping that your flight will land safely, help forge a sense of identity with others. When circumstances conspire to make us aware that we share a common experience or characteristic with others, a set of mental processes spontaneously kick into gear that causes us to feel like we are part of a group—nay, that causes us to actually *become* a group.

The consequences of this group-oriented psychology are profound. Our social identities provide a powerful basis for unity. But they can also be, as we saw with the Town of Bent Necks, a source of significant division.

A SOCIAL VACUUM

If one made an inventory of all the reasons groups come into conflict with one another, it would be a formidable list: competition over scarce resources, such as land, oil, food, treasure, or water. Battles over sacred beliefs, gods, and holy ground. Slights and insults long remembered. Glory-striving leaders seeking riches, fame, or better opinion polls. Misperceptions and misunderstandings. Fear of the unknown and fear of the other. Wars for status, for bragging rights, and for power.

14

It seems that intergroup divisions can be triggered over just about anything. Even, as it turns out, shoes. As we saw with the Town of Bent Necks, the basis for group identities and the divisions between them can be mundane from an outsider's perspective but deeply meaningful to group members themselves. Shoes might seem like a trivial thing for people to rally around, but to understand how such seemingly arbitrary things can become a powerful basis for identities, we need to tell you about what we consider to be among the most important studies in the history of psychology.

These are known as the "minimal-group studies," and they started as what was essentially just a control condition.

Many things can work in combination to make different groups dislike one another, discriminate, and even want to cause one another significant harm. Conflict over scarce resources may combine with negative stereotypes and differences in power. These might be further inflamed by a leader's divisive rhetoric and reinforced by memories of old battles from decades or even centuries ago. All of these factors and more can combine in unique ways to drive intergroup conflicts.

To get a handle on the underlying dynamics of intergroup relations, social scientists would like to be able to isolate these different factors and study them separately, much as a chemist isolates a compound to better understand its properties. However, it is very difficult to isolate a single component of a real-life conflict between, say, religious, ethnic, or political groups because they co-occur. These factors tend to come as a package.

In order to resolve this problem and understand what causes conflict, Henri Tajfel and his collaborators at the University of Bristol hit upon a brilliant idea. Chemists create airtight vacuums when they want to isolate a compound, and using that logic, Tajfel and his colleagues came up with a way to make a type of social vacuum. They created a situation in which all of the factors involved in intergroup conflict—stereotypes, resource disparities, insults, and so on—were stripped away, leaving only the most minimal version of an intergroup context. It's a situation involving two groups but without any of the ingredients that generally produce discrimination or conflict.

Having created a social vacuum by removing all these key factors, they could slowly start adding different ingredients into the situation to see what produced discrimination and conflict. Adding a splash of resource competition here, a drop of stereotyping there, and so on would allow them to study how each of these ingredients affects relations between groups.

To create a vacuum, the researchers could not use preexisting, real-life groups because they came with a certain amount of psychological baggage. Instead, they assigned participants to completely novel groups on the basis of arbitrary and essentially meaningless criteria.[3] Participants in one study were informed they were "overestimators" or "underestimators" based on how many dots they thought were displayed on an image. In another study, they were placed in groups based on their preference for the abstract art of either Paul Klee or Wassily Kandinsky. But things were not what they seemed. The people in the overestimator group did not really tend to overestimate the number of dots, and the members of the Klee fan group did not necessarily like *Twittering Machine* (yes, that is the actual name of a famous piece). In each case, the researchers had essentially flipped a coin and assigned people to groups based on chance. This ensured that their actual dot-estimation styles or artist preferences would have no bearing on how they treated in-group and out-group members.

Participants in these studies were then asked to allocate resources between members of their in-group (fellow Klee fans, say) and members of the out-group (those so-called Kandinsky fanatics). In several studies, participants divided money between an anonymous in-group member and an anonymous out-group member. The researchers took steps to ensure a social vacuum by keeping the situation as empty as possible. Participants had absolutely no inter-action with other members of either group. There was no period of getting to know one another, no chance to form personal bonds, and no competition over resources. It was simply us and them, two minimal groups.

Participants' decisions were not zero-sum. This point is important because it meant that giving more to one group did not have to mean giving less to the other. Finally, their decisions had no direct bearing on their own outcomes—they could not personally earn more or less by behaving in particular ways.

The researchers assumed this would make an excellent control condition. With all possible reasons for discriminating between the groups presumably eliminated, it seemed like a solid basis for inter-group harmony. Once this was established, they could then conduct future studies where they systematically added in the different in-gredients for intergroup conflict to find out exactly what mattered. But the results were startling, even to the researchers themselves.

People assigned to a minimal group, far from losing their inter-group bias, consistently discriminated in favor of their own group. If the coin flip had led them to believe they were Kandinsky fans, they gave more resources to a fellow Kandinsky fan than to a Klee admirer. And the opposite was true for supposed Klee enthusiasts.

Strikingly, people sometimes actually *maximized* the difference be-tween the groups. Given the choice, they would allocate less money to an in-group member if it meant that an out-group member got even less.

The researchers had stripped away stereotypes, resource conflict, status differences, and everything else they could think of. So what was left? What residue remained in the social vacuum that could possibly account for people showing such clear preferences for these most arbitrary, short-lived, and meaningless of groups?

The answer that came to Henri Tajfel and colleagues was *social identity*.[4] It seemed that the mere fact of being categorized as part

17

of one group rather than another was enough to link that group membership to a person's sense of self. Sitting there in the laboratory, people thought of themselves not as disinterested observers in a weird resource-allocation experiment but as members of a real social group with value and meaning. Even in a social vacuum, people shared a sense of identity with anonymous strangers—simply because they believed they were part of the same group. Motivated to possess an identity that was meaningful and of value, participants took the only course of action they had available in the situation to make that true: they allocated more resources to in-group than out-group members. They acted to ensure that their brand-new identity was a positive and a distinct one—and in doing so, they began to advance their group's interests even though there was no obvious benefit to themselves as individuals.

Variants of these experiments have been conducted around the globe to examine how a shared sense of "us" can affect all manner of psychological processes, including attention, perception, and memory, as well as emotions like empathy and schadenfreude, that naughty feeling of pleasure in other people's pain we sometimes get.

Subsequent research has found that much of the bias that is created when someone joins and identifies with a group—minimal or real—is better characterized as reflecting in-group love than out-group hate. People typically like their own groups more, but this doesn't necessarily mean they dislike or want to harm out-groups. When people in minimal groups are asked to deliver aversive outcomes to other people, for example, they show less of a preference for their own group—they don't particularly want to cause the out-group harm.[5] In our own studies with minimal groups, we have found that people automatically feel positively toward in-group members but feel neutral toward out-group members.[6] Of course, relations between groups can become hateful, especially when factors like demeaning stereotypes, inflammatory rhetoric, or resource competition enter the situation. We will discuss these group dynamics throughout the book and tell you more about our own research on minimal groups. We have found that assigning people to an arbitrary group can immediately affect patterns of brain activity, change how they look at others, and, at least momentarily, override racial biases. The minimal-group studies have inspired much of our work and fundamentally reshaped how we understand the nature of human identity. They have clarified to us that there is no true social vacuum. In many ways, the psychology of groups is the natural human condition.

SHIFTING IDENTITIES AND CHANGING GOALS

For as long as humans have been capable of self-reflection, they have thought about the nature of the self. What does it mean to have a self? What is its purpose? To the philosopher René Descartes, who was temporarily in doubt about the existence of all things, the self was a point of certainty from which he could reason everything else back into being: "I think, therefore I am." The philosopher Daniel Dennett has memorably described the self as the "center of narrative gravity." In other words, we are at the hearts of our own stories.

But the minimal-group studies reveal that the human sense of self—your gravitational center—does not stay in the same place. With the flip of a coin, people constructed entirely new identities in a matter of minutes. The sense of self moves about, shifting between different aspects of identity. And this movement has consequences for how you perceive and make sense of the world, as well as the choices you make.

Over the course of a few hours, the same person's identity—the sense of self that is active at a given moment—might shift from self as individual in the car fighting through traffic on the way to work to self as employee representing one's company on a conference

19

call to self as supporter of a political party arguing about the news on social media to self as sports fan watching a game on TV and, finally, to self as romantic partner at the end of the day. One person can hold all of these identities, and many more besides.

As the gravitational center of your self shifts, and as one identity or another is activated, the goals that motivate you and the people whose fates you are concerned with shift as well. More generally, as identity expands from an individual to a social or collective level of self, other people are brought within the sphere of your self-interest. *I* becomes *we*. *Me* becomes *us*. *Mine* becomes *ours*.

These motivational changes are beautifully illustrated by experiments conducted by social psychologists David De Cremer and Mark Van Vugt.[7] They started by classifying university students based on what is known as their "social value orientation." Social value orientation captures how much you tend to take your own and other people's interests into account when you make decisions. To measure your social value orientation, researchers ask you to imagine how you would divide different sums of money between yourself and someone else. Each time, you confront choices. Do you try to maximize your own earnings? Do you try to help your partner? Or would you prefer to widen the gap between yourself and the other person?

As an example, think about which of the following options you would choose. Option A gives you and your partner 500 points each. Option B gives you 560 points and your partner 300. Option C gives you 400 points and your partner 100. Which would you choose?

If you consistently choose distributions like option A, you have a *cooperative* or *pro-social orientation,* because the option provides an equal distribution of outcomes. If you prefer choices like option B, you have a more *individualistic orientation,* because you are maximizing your own outcomes irrespective of what other people are getting. Finally, if you are an option C kind of person, you have a *competitive orientation,* because this distribution maximizes the difference between your own and the other person's outcomes. This was the orientation that seemed to animate Adi and Rudi in the Town of Bent Necks, at least with respect to each other.

The researchers in this case lumped the individualists and competitors together into a single category that they called *pro-selfs* and compared them to the *pro-socials*. Having figured out the participants' social value orientations, the researchers designed an experiment to manipulate which aspect of participants' self-concepts was most salient or active in the moment. They did this by randomly assigning them to complete a task that highlighted each subject's identity as either a university student or an individual. The researchers then measured how much they were willing to contribute in an economic game to a group composed of fellow university students.

These economic games were structured so that choosing to do what was best for the group required a degree of personal sacrifice—opting to give more to the collective and keep a little less for themselves. Unsurprisingly, the people who were classified as pro-social were always fairly generous. They contributed to their group regardless of whether their identities as university students had been activated or not, donating real money roughly 90 percent of the time.

The people with a pro-self social value orientation were different. Predictably, they were less generous than the pro-socials when their individual identity had been highlighted. In this condition, they contributed to the group a mere 44 percent of the time. They were half as generous.

However, this pattern was completely changed among pro-selfs when their social identity as university students had been made salient. When their identity was temporarily defined by membership in a group, generosity among pro-selfs nearly doubled, and they gave to the group 79 percent of the time. They were nearly indistinguishable from people with a pro-social orientation.

The implications of this finding are profound. It is unlikely that the people with pro-self orientations had miraculously become less self-interested. Instead, their self-interested motives had *transformed* from their individual self to a group self. This is one of the tricks performed by social identity. It transforms goals and can make even selfish people behave in pro-social ways.

CONTAINING MULTITUDES

Do I contradict myself?
Very well, then I contradict myself
(I am large, I contain multitudes.)
    —Walt Whitman, "Song of Myself"

We are painting a picture of identity that is dynamic and multifaceted. People are often walking contradictions. They contain multitudes. But despite plenty of evidence that human identity is complex and changeable, this can still feel deeply counterintuitive. Our moment-to-moment experience tends to feel quite consistent and it can be hard to recognize, even in oneself, the flexibility of identity across time and place. Once, when one of us was talking about this in a class, a student exclaimed in frustration: "If what you're saying is right, how many selves do I have? Who on earth am I?"

So who on earth are we? How numerous are the multitudes within us?

Social psychologists use a technique known as the twenty-statements task to tap into different components of people's identities. It's very simple; all you have to do is complete the sentence "I am _____" twenty times.

Here is a sampling from our own lists:

Dom	Jay
A professor	A father
A father	A scientist
A husband	A Canadian
Intelligent	A son
Stressed out	A social neuroscientist
A social psychologist	An optimist
A music lover	A kid from Fox Creek
A redhead	A hockey goalie
A Pennsylvanian	A social media addict
An amateur cook	A politics junkie

If you write your own list, you might note several interesting things. First, it's usually not too hard to come up with twenty or so items that you consider self-defining. We found ourselves slowing down a bit toward the end, but many aspects of ourselves came readily to mind.

Second, most people's lists include things that can be lumped into certain categories. Some are clearly about an *individual level* of self. Stable personality traits such as *intelligent* and *optimist,* as well as more temporary states like *stressed out,* refer to aspects of the person as a unique entity. These are characteristics that differentiate one person from another.

Other components refer to a *relational level* of self. To be a *father* or *husband,* for example, is to be someone in relation to at least one other person, and it is your role in the relationship that defines that piece of your identity. And other components involve a *collective level* of self; social identities like *Pennsylvanian* and *social neuroscientist* define you as a member of a category that you feel is important to who you are.

There are other interesting features of these lists. Research suggests that people are more likely to incorporate something into their identity if it is distinct and differentiating.[8] Red hair occurs naturally in only about 2 percent of the population, so it's more likely that Dominic would write *redhead* on his list of self-defining attributes than that Jay would write *brunet*. Some attributes can belong to more than one level of identity. Identifying yourself as a redhead means viewing your hair color as a trait that differentiates you from others. But hair color can also serve as a basis for social categorization, a way of dividing the world into groups. Indeed, there are stereotypes about redheads as a category. As was said of Anne of Green Gables, perhaps the world's most famous fictional redhead, "Her temper matches her hair."[9] Understanding themselves to be a distinct group, redheads have even organized their own festivals, online communities, and dating websites.

The fact is that individual aspects of identity are hard to separate from social aspects of identity. This is true in at least two additional ways. First, many personal traits are inherently relative and gain meaning only in comparison to others. To self-define as intelligent, for example, is to consider oneself smarter than other people; to self-define as an optimist is to see oneself as more positively expectant than others. Importantly, the people against whom you assess yourself are generally people you consider to be relevant targets for comparison, and these are much more likely to be in-group rather than out-group members.

Second, the social groups we belong to shape the very experience of what it is to be an individual. The ways in which you strive to be an independent self are influenced by the norms of the groups you identify with. Norms are the accepted standards of behavior within social groups and influence how you behave. The more that someone identifies with a group, the more strongly he or she will tend to conform to that group's norms. In other words, strongly identified members are more likely than weakly identified members to think, feel, and act similarly to most other people in their group.

People from more collectivist cultures might be nodding along, but if you are from an individualistic culture, you might be reading this with some skepticism. You likely don't think of yourself as a conformist. However, it turns out that this is also a social norm!

Some groups have individualistic norms. For example, the American identity has a strong independent streak, emphasizing the importance of personal autonomy, responsibility, and individual rights and deemphasizing the importance of consensus and cohesion. What does this mean for strongly identified Americans? Their level of identification should lead them to conform more to the norms of the group, making them strive to be even more individualistic.

Does this mean that American individualism is really a type of conformity? The results of research by Jolanda Jetten at the University of Queensland and her colleagues suggest that indeed it is.[10] In one study, they found that strongly identified Americans expressed higher levels of individualism than weakly identified Americans. Thus, Americans who express their individualism are, in fact, conformists to a very strong social norm.

American norms create, in the immortal words of art critic Harold Rosenberg, a "herd of independent minds." We call it the *independence paradox*—that people who strive for independence are often doing it to fit in! In contrast, in Jetten's research strongly identified Indonesians, members of a nation with more collectivistic norms, expressed higher levels of collectivism than weakly identified Indonesians.

Lest you think this is purely an issue of national culture, there is plenty of variation within nations as well. When we worked at Ohio State, we noted that the undergraduates were obsessed with fitting in, and a great many wore scarlet and gray, the school colors, with pride. And on game days, it wasn't only the students garbed in scarlet and gray—it was the whole city of Columbus. When the Buck-eyes played football, more than a hundred thousand people would pack the stadium and chant in unison to traditional fight songs. As the team marched toward the national championship during our first year in Ohio, the entire city was immersed in identity rituals.

It was a rousing and fascinating anthropological experience for two lads coming from the University of Toronto, where the football team had recently set a national record by losing its forty-ninth game in a row. But when we moved to our current jobs at Lehigh University (Dominic) and New York University (Jay), the norms were radically different. It is rare to see an NYU student wearing the school colors, and the value these students cherish more than any other is "being interesting." To them, blending in means standing out.

Of course, people know different universities offer different cultures. This helps people to sort themselves, opting to join different types of communities depending on the local norms and educational environment. Applicants who have a strong desire to fit in with a highly cohesive community will likely have a better experience at Ohio State than at Lehigh. Applicants who have a strong desire to cultivate and embody a striking individuality will likely have a better experience at NYU than at Ohio State. It is also the case that after arriving on campus, students may find their identities changing to align more closely with their university's social norms.

Similar dynamics had played out in our graduate-student office at the University of Toronto. While Jay was fond of wearing flip-flops and ironic T-shirts, Dominic emulated professors a few years his senior and started showing up to work in a suit jacket. Before long, Jay found himself drawn to a brown corduroy blazer with elbow patches. While this shift seemed like the natural next step in Jay's growing sense of fashion, the reality is that it likely stemmed from his more dapper office mate and identification with the professors in his department. This is precisely how identity and norms shape our decisions. When Jay moved to Ohio State, and Dom followed a few months later, Dom was mortified to discover that everyone in Columbus thought he was emulating Jay! More troubling still, Jay did nothing to correct this misperception.

Hazel Marcus at Stanford University and her colleagues have studied differences in these sorts of norms between Americans who live in urban versus rural settings.[11] In many big cities, people would be mortified if their best friends bought the same outfits or decorated their apartments in exactly the same way. Too much similarity impinges on their individualism. But in rural locations, people are more likely to believe that imitation is the sincerest form of flattery and take pleasure in sharing common experiences with their friends. This is why hipsters, obsessed with authenticity and uniqueness, cluster in gentrified urban neighborhoods, while odd deviations from the norm can lead to teasing or ostracism in more traditional rural communities.

One of the most important functions of groups is their ability to coordinate the behaviors and activities of many people at once. Like our friends the honeybees and our enemies the termites, humans are a hyper-social species, living together in collectives that range from the small scale (couples and families) to the truly massive (countries with hundreds of millions of citizens). Unlike beehives and termite colonies, however, the groups, organizations, and societies we build are endlessly evolving, allowing us to innovate, build new institutions, adapt to ever-changing environments, and benefit from the tremendous advantages of working together.

A great deal of this coordination is accomplished via conformity to norms. Conformity has been observed in every domain of life where researchers have looked for it. Experiments have revealed conformity in fashion, political and musical preferences, moral values, eating and drinking behaviors, sexual practices, social attitudes, cooperation, and conflict. What people think, feel, and do is influenced, often to a startling degree, by what they believe everyone else is thinking, feeling, and doing. And because they are bound to groups and identities, the particular norms that guide people at any given moment can vary depending on which parts of themselves are the most salient and active.

ARE BANKERS DISHONEST?

Bankers, like lawyers and politicians, don't have the best reputation when it comes to honesty. Gallup polling in 2019, for example, found that 20 percent of people rated bankers' honesty and ethics as low or very low, compared to just 3 percent for nurses and 6 percent for dentists.[12] Public perception of bankers' integrity worsened after the 2008 financial crisis and never fully recovered. Bankers were rated as having poor ethics by 55 percent of respondents, although they still had a better reputation than members of the U.S. Congress.

To examine how much the stereotype of bankers matches the reality of their behavior, economists at the University of Zurich—near the heart of one of the world's largest banking centers—devised a clever experiment.[13] They asked bankers at an international firm to flip a coin ten times and record how often it came up heads and how often it came up tails. The bankers were told in advance that one type of outcome—either heads or tails—would be rewarded. So, for example, if heads were rewarded, they would receive the equivalent of about twenty dollars for every time the coin came up heads and nothing when it came up tails. To increase the stakes, bankers were informed that they would receive their winnings *only if* their total exceeded an amount won by a randomly selected participant in another study.

Critically, the bankers made their coin tosses in private, away from the prying eyes of the experimenter. They could, therefore, report any number of heads or tails they wanted, and no one would be the wiser. The incentives to cheat were strong, putting the bankers' honesty firmly to the test.

Before the bankers began the coin-tossing task, half of them were reminded of their professional identity with questions like "At what bank are you currently working?" Being asked about their occupation was expected to activate this aspect of their identity, making it highly salient prior to tossing the coin. In contrast, the other half of the bankers were asked questions that had nothing to do with their job, like "How many hours a week do you watch television?" This would get them thinking about their personal identity or other identities outside of work.

We don't know how many heads or tails any particular banker actually got; the outcomes really were private. But we do know that 50 percent of the time a coin is flipped, it should come up heads. By comparing how close the reported numbers of heads and tails in each condition were to what would be expected by chance, the researchers could determine whether bankers in one condition were more likely to cheat than bankers in the other condition.

Bankers asked about their television habits and other mundane aspects of their lives did not appear to cheat. On average, they reported flipping their coins to the advantageous side 51.6 percent of the time—which was not statistically different from chance. However, cheating was elevated among bankers reminded of their occupational identity! This group of bankers reported securing advantageous coin flips 58.2 percent of the time.

Are bankers dishonest? The answer, it appears, is that it depends on whether the bankers in question are thinking about themselves as bankers! Bankers, like everyone else, contain multitudes.

What this further suggests is that the question "Are bankers dishonest?" is not actually very meaningful. Whether one's identity as a banker will influence one's honesty depends on the norms of the banking community with which one identifies—norms that can differ between groups and presumably change over time.

This may be why a recent paper that looked at how activating occupational identities influenced honesty among bankers in the

Middle East and in Asia did not find the same effect.[14] The norms of banks in these locations—and certainly the norms of the broader cultures in which they operate—are likely different from those in the original study.[15] There may also be differences among types of bankers; while those in the original study were primarily involved in investment and trading, those in the second were commercial bankers who primarily dealt with loans.

ON REPLICATION

Concerns that previously published findings cannot be replicated have grown considerably in psychology—and, indeed, many scientific fields—over the past few years, leading to what some have called a "reproducibility crisis." As the saga of the banker studies highlights, making sense of what it means when a previous finding is not replicated is not always straightforward. Perhaps the original finding wasn't real. Maybe it was a statistical fluke (the chances of which can be increased with sample sizes that are too small), an artifact of dodgy data handling, or, in rare cases, outright fraud. In many other cases, if research finds a pattern of behavior in one context and not in another, it might reflect meaningful variation in factors that alter the results. This is one of the primary interests of social and cultural psychology. In the case of the banker studies, we think that there is a sound reason to suspect that different norms explain why some banker identities increase dishonesty while others do not. But the truth is that without further research, we don't know for sure.

For all of the research we talk about in this book, there is an important distinction to be made between findings from specific studies and the broader identity principles that they illuminate. In this case, there is a massive literature demonstrating that people are highly influenced by group norms, some of which we will talk about more deeply in later chapters. So if you have children or friends who work in banking, you shouldn't assume based on the study we described that they are ethically compromised in the workplace. You should, however, be interested in what sorts of norms their employers hold. And if you personally are thinking of taking a job in a bank—or anywhere else—we think that you should be especially interested in what the local norms are, because they will likely exert an important influence on your behavior and your life.

In this book, we have tried to focus on findings in which we have high levels of confidence. But the underlying principles of identity that this book is about are grounded in many more studies than we have room to discuss. The principles are supported by extensive lines of research conducted by multiple laboratories, often over many years. Not everything is settled, of course, and where ideas have evolved, controversies continue, and questions remain, we will talk about them. Indeed, how scientific understanding evolves over time is one of the most interesting parts of the story!

PRINCIPLES OF IDENTITY

This chapter lays out several key lessons about identities and the roles they play in people's lives. First, the groups people belong to are often fundamental to their sense of self and understanding of who they are. Second, people have a remarkable readiness to find collective solidarity with others and generate, even if only temporarily, a sense of identity based on common experiences, shared characteristics, and even random assignment to a new group. Third, when a particular social identity is salient and active, it can have a profound effect on people's goals, emotions, and behaviors. Fourth, most people are quite likely to conform to the norms associated with an active identity and try to act in ways that they believe will advance its interests, making personal sacrifices if necessary.

A great number of good things result when we create and share social identities with others. But there is another side to this: cooperation and generosity are bound by our identities. For every in-group, there is usually an out-group. Social identities can make people want to help members of their own groups, but it can also make them want to harm—or at least avoid helping—people who belong to other groups.

Speaking of conflict between groups, in this book we will talk quite a lot about political identities. In many nations around the world, political polarization or sectarian conflict is causing massive social strife. Politics in many places have become remarkably toxic.

When relations between groups harden and we start to see "our" interests as fundamentally opposed to "their" interests, the natural positive emotions and empathy we feel toward our own groups can shift in a dangerous direction. We start to think that we're not only good but that we're *inherently* good. And if that's true, then *they* must be intrinsically bad and should be opposed at all costs. Issues are moralized in ways that favor our point of view. We become less tolerant of dissent and vigilant against any deviance that threatens to dilute the all-important boundary between us and them. We see enemies without and within. We begin to believe that when it comes to pursuing our group's interests, any means justifies the ends. And when we do commit harm against others, it is often because we think it is pursuant to a larger, virtuous goal.

Many people don't realize how much competition relies on cooperation. When people play checkers or hockey or compete for a promotion, they implicitly agree to abide by a shared and mutually agreed upon set of rules. In politics too there are rules, written in constitutions and carved out by tradition and precedent. These rules, embodied by political institutions, allow rivals to engage in fierce debate and hash things out without resorting to bloodshed.

Effective institutions that provide fair rules and accountability are among the most important social goods a human society can provide. And these institutions work as long as enough people believe in them, as long as they believe that there is something larger and ultimately more important than winning the next election. Toxic politics are especially dangerous when they undermine these beliefs. Things can get truly ugly when the loss of any sense of shared identity as citizens combines with a group's belief in its own righteousness, leading its members to think that playing by the rules is foolish or that the other side must be stopped at all costs.

We believe that these toxic patterns are products of standard group and identity dynamics but that these bad outcomes are by no means inevitable. Intergroup interactions and politics do not have to be this way. Understanding how identity works can help us make sense of what's going on and, perhaps, figure out how we can get out of this mess.

Although our social identities can be powerful forces in our lives, we nevertheless have agency and some level of control over them. All people belong to some categories that they don't especially value or identify with, even if others do. For this reason, when we as researchers study people's social identities, we don't assume that everyone in a category, whether it's gender, race, occupation, religion, or nationality (just to name a few), is equally identified with it. Instead, we often measure how much each person identifies with the group. We might ask people to rate how proud they are to belong to the group and how central it is to their sense of self.

Of course, people don't have full control over which groups they belong to, but they often have the capacity to choose which ones they embrace as identities. When you choose a college or a career, support a sports team, or register with a political party, you are actively selecting a certain identity. Likewise, if you abandon a party, quit a job, or even stop being a smoker, you are letting go of an identity. Given how much of people's emotions, beliefs, and behaviors are wrapped up in their social identities, the agency to choose which ones they care about, which ones will animate their choices, and which ones will define their relationship to the world is critically important. Indeed, these might be among the most important decisions anyone makes in life.

People also exert their agency when they dissent from group norms or take a more active role in leadership. Identity is central to both of these tasks. As we will explain, people are more willing to dissent if they care deeply about a group, and leaders are more effective when they can generate a shared sense of identity among their followers.

The premise at the heart of our book is that knowing how identities work can give us more control over their influence. As we said before, understanding social identity allows us to transition from asking "Who am I?" to figuring out "Who do I want to be?"

WHAT COMES NEXT?

The first chapters of this book look at how social identities shape how we experience the world and the decisions we make. Chapters 2, 3, and 4 describe how social identities provide the lenses through which we perceive events and how they influence some of our most important beliefs. Together, we will explore the role of identity in political partisanship, how new technologies, including social media, have made that partisanship worse, and potential solutions for bridging divides. In chapter 5, we examine why people value certain social identities more than others and how these identities imbue relevant symbols and objects with value.

Social identities always exist in intergroup contexts; we often exhibit biases in favor of our own groups and to the detriment of others. In chapter 6, we will examine the nature of biases—both implicit and explicit—and discuss how they are often grounded in long histories of oppression and institutional structures. Understanding how social identities work can offer solutions for reducing bias, but tackling systemic discrimination requires a broader scale of action.

Subsequent chapters will then examine how identities underlie collective action. In chapter 7, we discuss how social identities arise in response to adversity and provide a foundation for solidarity in pursuit of social change. In chapter 8, we will explore how insiders change their groups from within, how identity dynamics influence who dissents, and how groups can capitalize on a diversity of perspectives. Chapter 9 will explain the critical role that leaders play in all of these domains. We will examine how effective leaders seek to meet group members' identity needs, helping them figure out who they are and where they are going. The tools of identity leadership can be used for good or for evil.

Finally, in chapter 10, we speculate on what might lie in store for group life. We will focus on the challenges that humanity confronts regarding rising inequality, climate change, and threats to democracy. Effectively grappling with these issues hinges on understanding the role of identity.

Starting in chapter 2, we will delve into how identities alter perceptions, affecting how we filter and make sense of information in the world around us. Identities provide us with lenses through which we experience the world and make meaning, but they can also misdirect our attention and bias our judgments.

CHAPTER 2

THE LENS OF IDENTITY

An audience of four hundred million sat glued to their seats as the final game of the 1966 FIFA World Cup moved into overtime. With the world's most coveted championship trophy on the line, England and West Germany were deadlocked, two to two. More than ten nail-biting minutes of extra time had elapsed when English player Alan Ball passed the ball to Geoff Hurst, a lanky striker from Lancashire.

Hurst shot the ball off his right foot toward the goal as he fell to the ground. The ball edged over the outstretched fingertips of the German keeper, struck the bottom of the crossbar, ricocheted toward the goal line, and was cleared away by West German defenders.

The world championship rested on what had happened during that split second.

The English players, believing they had won the game, began to celebrate. The crowd roared! Yet Swiss referee Gottfried Dienst was not sure that England had actually scored. At the time, Dienst was considered the best referee in the world. Uncertain, he consulted with his assistant before making the critical decision: the ball had crossed the line. Goal!

Video footage would ultimately show that the ball had not, in fact, crossed the line. England should not have won the 1966 World

Cup 4–2—at least, not with that score line. Yet the English player closest to the ball, Roger Hunt, swore that he had seen the ball cross the line and enter the net. Surely he must have seen it, otherwise he would have moved to tap it in rather than turning away to celebrate.

He saw what he wanted to see.

This situation might seem like a rarity. How often is the most widely viewed athletic contest in the world determined by such a contentious play? Yet sports fans everywhere constantly find themselves at odds with referees, umpires, and judges. The problem is that many fans are so affected by their own team identities that they feel that everyone else's decision-making is hopelessly biased—especially when the situation is ambiguous.

Research on this issue began following a football game played by two Ivy League teams at Palmer Stadium in Princeton, New Jersey, on a brisk Saturday afternoon in late November 1951. It was the last game of the season, and the Princeton University Tigers were trying to finish the year undefeated by beating the Dartmouth University Indians.

It quickly became clear that this was going to be a rough game. Players collided, anger rose, and violence swiftly escalated. Before long, Princeton's brilliant All-American quarterback Dick Kazmaier left the field with a broken nose. (He would later win the Heisman Trophy, which is awarded annually to the best player in college football, by the largest vote margin in history.) Losing their superstar infuriated the Princeton players. They retaliated. And in the third quarter, a Dartmouth player was carried off the field with a broken leg.

Princeton won the game thirteen to nothing. But that wasn't the end of the story.

The blame game started immediately. The Princeton student newspaper called the game a "disgusting exhibition" and reported that the "blame must be laid primarily on Dartmouth's doorstep." The Dartmouth student paper staff, however, saw it very differently.

They alleged that Princeton coach Charlie Caldwell had "instilled the old see-what-they-did-go-get-them attitude" in his players.

This feisty back-and-forth inspired psychologists at Dartmouth and Princeton to join forces to understand how it was that members of their exclusive colleges could disagree so fiercely about the objective facts of the game. They administered a questionnaire to Dartmouth and Princeton students a week after the game.[1] Just like the journalists from their college newspapers, Princeton and Dartmouth students had radically different interpretations of the game. Overall, one hundred twenty-two students claimed that the other team had started the rough play, and only two believed that their own team had initiated it!

Let us say that again: 122 to 2. A nearly unanimous verdict that it was the other guys' fault.

Because these disagreements could be chalked up to errors of memory or exposure to the biased newspaper reports, the researchers brought in a new batch of students from each school and showed them footage from the game. They recorded these students' responses as they watched the game unfold before their eyes. Maybe the video would provide a reality check.

Even though they were all looking at the same visual evidence, students from the two colleges continued to disagree about the facts of the game. Princeton students claimed that the Dartmouth players committed more than twice as many infractions as the Princeton players had; Dartmouth students claimed that the number of infractions was nearly identical for both teams. Even as they all watched the same video, students at each university still seemed to see very different things.

In case you are tempted to dismiss this as just the delusions of some college students, consider the telegram that a Dartmouth alumnus in Ohio sent to his alma mater. He had received footage of the game from friends, a group of Princeton alumni, who told him all about the dastardly behavior of his beloved Dartmouth team. But upon watching the footage, he couldn't see the fouls they had told him about and was genuinely puzzled.

Planning to show a tape of the game at an upcoming alumni event, he sent a telegram to Dartmouth administrators. "Preview of Princeton movies indicates considerable cutting of important part STOP please wire explanation and possibly air mail missing part before showing scheduled for January 25 STOP we have splicing equipment."

He assumed that some of the terrible fouls he'd heard about from his Princeton friends must have been cut from the tape!

Writing over sixty years ago, the researchers concluded, "the 'same' sensory impingements emanating from the football field, transmitted through the visual mechanism to the brain, also obviously gave rise to different experiences in different people." In other words, the fans were biased—they saw the game through the lens of their identification with the team, detecting every violation committed by their opponents but turning a blind eye to infractions by their own players.

This study reveals something important about human perception: we are often driven by our identities to interpret the world in a certain way. In the next chapter, we will discuss how this plays out when it comes to our beliefs about the world. Here, we see that it extends even to perceptual judgments—what we see, hear, taste, and smell.

In the course of any game, there are dozens, if not hundreds, of ambiguous events that are open to interpretation through the lens of one's identity. Modern advances in refereeing and technology now allow for instant replays to help sort out these ambiguous situations. But the impact of identity on judgment goes well beyond the sports stadium to domains of life where instant replay cannot offer a correction for our judgments.

For the past decade, the two of us have examined how group identities—ranging from sports teams to political parties to nations—

can profoundly influence how people interpret the world around them. These dynamics play out everywhere—at the dinner table and in the criminal justice system. And while identities can heighten our senses, causing us to better savor the smell of chocolate or crave the taste of savory grits, they can also impair our ability to perceive things accurately or fairly. Much of this is happening outside our awareness. And few, if any, of us are immune.

IDENTITY-COLORED GLASSES

> We don't see things as they are; we see them
> as we are.
> —Anaïs Nin, *Seduction of the Minotaur*

Every moment in the day, there is more information reaching your sensory organs than can possibly be consciously processed. Attention enables your nervous system to select a portion of what is (hopefully) the most relevant information in order to process it more deeply. A great deal of information filtering occurs before people become consciously aware that something—a movement, a sound, the emission of a scent—has happened. Having a system for sorting the sensory wheat from the chaff is more than useful, it is essential.

A classic example of this is known as the "cocktail party effect."[2] At any large gathering, the buzzing of music and conversation resides mainly in the background as you pay attention to the person you're talking to. Your brain filters out the noise to allow you to focus on whatever fascinating story or gossip your friend is relaying.

Now, what happens if someone mentions your name in a conversation across the room? If you are like most people, hearing your name breaks through the background noise and shifts your attention. Suddenly you are all ears, attuned to what is being said about you. Are they speaking kindly or sharing an embarrassing anecdote?

This cocktail party effect occurs because your brain is *not* ignoring everything in the background. While you were chatting away, your unconscious mind was monitoring the surrounding conversations in case something relevant happened. Someone saying your name to other people, of course, is just about the most relevant thing that can happen!

How attention works is very complex, but you can think about what catches people's attention as coming in two different forms. Some things capture attention because they are salient in the environment. Sudden movements, strange noises, beautiful or noxious things, and your own name—all of these warrant your attention so that you can react to them appropriately. This type of orienting of attention is sometimes described as "bottom-up" processing.

Other things, however, capture your attention because you are already on the lookout for them. Things that you expect, want, or need tend to receive more attention because your brain has already decided that they are relevant. When you are looking for your car keys, for example, you will probably find your eyes drawn to everything small and shiny as your visual system seeks out the object you urgently need. This type of attentional orienting is known as "top-down" processing. Goals, needs, desires, and, yes, identities change what your sensory system is focused on.

When you adopt an identity, it is as if you put on a pair of glasses that filter your view of the world.[3] Identity helps you grapple with the vast amount of information continually bombarding your senses. It tells you what is important, where to look, when to listen, and perhaps even what to taste.

Once you join a group, you gain insight into what "we" (the members of the group) consider important and, therefore, what you can safely ignore. And this works well, for the most part. On the job, for example, you probably pay extra attention to your boss, attend the right workshops, and figure out how to navigate office politics. You learn to ignore certain kinds of e-mails, large meetings, and work events that suck your time and energy.

At the end of the day, you go home and put on a different lens to negotiate your family obligations, noisy neighbors, and friendships at the local pub. This is one of the most useful elements of identity. Just as people can switch from sunglasses to regular glasses when they enter a dark building or put on reading glasses in front of the computer, they can switch identities as they move from one situation to the next.

People possess different identities, and they shift how they perceive the world as different aspects of their selves are activated. For bicultural individuals, this effect may be even more profound. For people with more than one cultural or ethnic identity, different situations can activate distinct parts of themselves that then influence how they think about and perceive the people around them.

Cultural neuroscientist Joan Chiao and her colleagues have conducted fascinating research on this phenomenon.[4] In one experiment, she had Black, White, and biracial participants (individuals who had a White and a Black parent) complete a visual attention task. On each trial, participants were presented with up to eight faces for half a second. Sometimes their job was to quickly determine if there was a single Black face among a crowd of White faces. On other trials, they had to determine if there was a single White face among a crowd of Black faces.

Chiao and colleagues found that every group of participants was faster to visually identify Black faces among White crowds than White faces among Black crowds. However, there were two interesting findings that revealed how racial identity shaped visual attention. The first was that Black participants were faster than White participants at identifying Black faces in a crowd. They could spot an in-group member in a heartbeat.

The second striking thing was what happened among biracial

42

individuals. What we did not mention earlier was that before starting the visual attention task, these participants had been asked to write a short essay about the ethnic identity of one of their parents. This task was designed to activate one or the other of their cultural identities. And it changed how they reacted to the visual displays.

When bicultural participants' White ethnic identity was activated, their patterns of visual attention looked almost identical to the White participants'. But when their Black ethnic identity was activated, their patterns of visual attention looked almost identical to the Black participants'. In other words, their attentional system had shifted in line with whichever identity was active at that moment.

For humans, vision is usually the most powerful sense. For dogs, it's smell; for bats, sound. But when it comes to identity, other sensations can be particularly potent and evocative: The smell of your grandmother's cooking or the specific scent of a location. The sound of a particular language or a song learned in childhood. The tastes of your culture's time-honored, traditional foods.

Indeed, there appears to be a profound connection between food and identity. As the late chef and author Anthony Bourdain put it in an interview for *Slate*, "Food is everything we are. It's an extension of nationalist feeling, ethnic feeling, your personal history, your province, your region, your tribe, your grandma. It's inseparable from those from the get-go."

THE TASTE OF IDENTITY

In the 1992 movie *My Cousin Vinny*, Joe Pesci plays a New York City lawyer defending his cousin, who is on trial for a murder he did not commit. Dislocated to Alabama, this brash Italian American from the Big Apple tries to navigate the culture of the rural American South.

In a key scene, Pesci goes to a local diner and learns that grits, made from boiled cornmeal, are a big part of Southern identity.

Cooking grits properly takes twenty minutes, and it's a matter of Southern pride not to use the instant version.

Soon after, Pesci's character begins questioning one of the prosecution's witnesses, a Southerner by the name of Mr. Tipton. Tipton says that he was just starting to make his breakfast when he saw Vinny's cousin enter a store, and five minutes later, as Tipton was about to eat his breakfast, he heard a gunshot.

What did Tipton have for breakfast? Vinny wants to know. Eggs and grits, Tipton tells him. Vinny, with his newfound knowledge of Southern cooking, knows old-fashioned grits don't cook that fast, so he asks Tipton if he made *instant* grits for breakfast. This is a major insult, an affront to Tipton's Southern pride! At this moment, the witness has to admit either that his testimony was faulty or that he has betrayed his Southern heritage with an inferior form of grits.

The life of an innocent man hangs in the balance.

In front of the judge and a courtroom packed with members of his community, the witness decides he must defend his Southern identity even if it reveals that his timeline of events cannot be trusted. Tipton aggressively announces, "No self-respectin' Southerner uses instant grits. I take pride in my grits."

Would someone admit to false testimony just to defend his or her grits? Maybe not. But this was never about the grits; it was about identity. And because cultural traditions are often tightly interwoven with eating, there is a deep connection for many people between their identities and their food.

People travel the world to try exotic cuisines, but even a tour around a single country can reveal a vast multiplicity of tastes, textures, ingredients, and culinary traditions. In the United States, there are big differences in the culinary preferences of different regions. New Yorkers enjoy what they believe is the best pizza in the country, folks from Philadelphia savor their famous cheesesteaks, Californians are stereotyped for munching on avocado toast, and the South is known for grits, black-eyed peas, and delicious barbecue.

Drawing inspiration from *My Cousin Vinny*, we decided to study the links between Southern identity and people's experiences of food. How deeply are preferences for grits woven into Southern identity? We wondered whether reminding people about their Southern identity would make them crave the foods associated with their traditions.

In a series of experiments led by Leor Hackel, we recruited more than two hundred fifty Southerners to tell us about their identity and their food preferences.[5] The first thing we noticed was that our sample of Southerners varied widely in terms of how much they identified with the South. While many people reported that it was a central part of their identity, just as many felt little or no connection to the region. (As we discussed in chapter 1, this sort of variation is common within groups. For instance, some of our students deeply identify with their university. They wear the school colors, attend college sports, and talk about the school with incredible pride. But other students are ambivalent about their school or even actively disengaged from the community.)

After we had the Southerners tell us about their connection to the South, we asked them to rate a number of foods—from fried catfish to black-eyed peas—on how closely they were connected to Southern identity and how much they felt like eating each one. We wanted to see if there was a connection between the strength of their identity and how much they enjoyed Southern foods compared to foods from outside the region.

As we'd predicted, people's degree of identification with the South was clearly associated with a preference for Southern cuisine. It wasn't enough to come from the South—it was identification with the South that mattered when it came to food preferences. And, naturally, these proud Southerners had less interest in pizza, tuna sandwiches, and other food from other places. Identity matters when it comes to food preferences; it gives the food an emotional resonance that goes beyond the calories.

But as we have seen throughout, identities are not a stable or static thing. People from the South always have this cultural heritage, but that doesn't mean this aspect of the self is active or in play at every moment. Like the bankers who behaved more dishonestly when their banker identities were activated, Southerners, we suspected, would be more Southern in their culinary tastes when this identity was primed *and* they actually cared about the identity.

In a second study with a new set of people, we activated the subjects' Southern identity by having half of them describe two things that Southerners do often, two things they do well, and four traits associated with Southerners—two positive and two negative. The other half were asked to describe things they do as individuals and positive and negative traits they would ascribe to themselves. These questions were designed to activate either their Southern identity or their personal identity so we could see whether this would change their food preferences.

It was only after their Southern identity was brought to the front of their minds that Southerners preferred the taste of grits, collard greens, and other Southern delicacies more than those who had had their personal identity activated. When people were encouraged to think of themselves as individuals and focus on their own personality traits, their taste for Southern cuisine was unrelated to their Southern identity.

We found similar results when we took our project to an outdoor market in Ottawa, the capital city of Canada.[6] We teamed up with our colleague Michael Wohl, a psychology professor at Carleton University, who set up a booth in the ByWard Market—one of the oldest public markets in the country—and offered passersby the opportunity to compare the sweet tastes of fresh honey and maple syrup.

While both are sugary and sticky, only maple syrup is a symbol of Canadian identity. The Maple Leaf is, of course, displayed prominently on the center of the national flag, and Canada even has a

46

national strategic reserve of maple syrup in case of an emergency shortage (no kidding). Like hockey and beavers, maple syrup is considered a national treasure.

When our sample of Canadians did the taste test, they responded in much the same way that their neighbors in the American South had: they preferred the food associated with their heritage (maple syrup in this case), but only when we had activated their Canadian identity first. Thinking about Canadian identity whet their appetite for delicious maple syrup but not honey.

Our studies suggest that activating an identity can influence the sort of foods that people crave. Perhaps this is why many restaurants offering culturally specific cuisines strive to create an authentic ambience. It may be that adorning the walls of a Greek restaurant with images of the Parthenon or playing K-pop hits at a Korean barbecue place helps deepen a desire for dishes associated with those cultures.

This is not limited to adults (or K-pop stans); kids have social identities too and use similar cues to guide their eating. One series of studies with young children found that kids as young as one year old used social identity cues to determine what to eat. When the infants were given a choice between two foods, they chose the one endorsed by someone who spoke their native language and turned up their noses at the one that had been endorsed by someone speaking a foreign language.[7]

From a very young age, humans are sensitive to cues about identity, and language appears to be one of the most powerful signals of shared connection. This is a striking finding because kids at the age of one can hardly be described as foodies and they have to look to adults for guidance about what to eat. Yet they seem to intuit a connection between food and identity before they understand a great many other things.

This research reveals how identity shapes our food preferences and probably our diets. But it only scratches the surface of how different identities shape the way people experience the world. We believe that these preferences extend beyond mere cravings and can actually shape basic perceptions more directly, even influencing the sense of smell.

SMELLS LIKE CHOCOLATE

To investigate deeper effects of identity, we conducted a series of studies at the University of Geneva in Switzerland with our colleague Géraldine Coppin.[8] We wanted to investigate how identity shapes how people smell the world around them using one of our own guilty pleasures—chocolate (although Dom prefers his dark, while Jay is a fan of smoother milk varieties).

Switzerland is famous for its banks, stunning alps, multi-tooled army knives, and some of the world's best chocolatiers. To create the stimuli for this experiment, we worked with chemists to create scented felt-tip markers (like the fruit-scented markers kids use) that smelled like delicious Swiss chocolate.

We had Swiss as well as non-Swiss citizens, all students at the same university in Geneva, come into the lab. Just as with our studies on Southern food and maple syrup, we randomly selected a subset of our participants and reminded them of their Swiss identities. Others were reminded of their personal identities. We then had them smell the chocolate-scented markers twenty times and we recorded how intensely they detected the smell each time. This allowed us to look at the effect of identity on smell over time.

To provide a control condition, we used markers that smelled like buttery popcorn. Both scents were of easily recognized foods. But while people might associate the smell of popcorn with going to the movies, we assumed that the scent of chocolate would have a strong association with Swiss identity. We expected that only the scent of chocolate would resonate with our Swiss participants, especially when they were thinking about the world through the lens of their Swiss identity.

It is normal in experiments like this for people to find all smells intense at first, but due to a process known as habituation, they detect them less and less intensely over time. You have probably had the experience of walking into a bakery and being hit by an over-whelming aroma of freshly baked bread or into an office where all you can smell is someone's perfume. After a few minutes, though, the smell recedes and becomes part of the background. It is still detectable if you think about it but it's no longer overpowering. Your sensory system has adapted.

The same thing happened when the people in our study smelled the popcorn. At first, this smell was intense, but eventually it faded. In fact, in almost every condition of our experiment, including the one with the chocolate-scented marker, people exhibited habitua-tion. There was, however, one striking exception: Swiss citizens who had been reminded of their Swiss identity did *not* habituate to the smell of chocolate. This sweet smell remained strong to them even after the twentieth trial. It was an aromatic reminder of their iden-tity. Thinking about things like the beautiful Swiss Alps, high-end watches, and their world-famous banking system appeared to alter their sensitivity to chocolate.

Chocolate has, for most people anyway, a delightful, enticing scent. But odors range from the tantalizing to the terrible. Could social identities influence the experience of some of life's more ghastly smells as well? A team of researchers in the United Kingdom, led by Stephen Reicher, decided to find out.[9]

The materials they used in this study certainly rank among the more unusual. They asked a male research assistant to wear the same T-shirt for a week, including while he engaged in exercise and even while he slept. After being worn for a week, the shirt, it's safe to say, was fairly pungent. It was then carefully sealed in an airtight container to maintain the odor until the study was ready to commence.

A while later, unsuspecting and unfortunate students from the

University of Sussex were asked if they would mind taking a whiff of the odorous garment. (Imagine showing up for a study and being asked to sniff someone else's dirty laundry.) After smelling the shirt, they rated their level of disgust. Naturally, most reported feeling a great deal of it.

But the researchers used a clever trick to see if social identity might influence how people respond to nasty odors. All of the participants had to smell the stinky shirt, which bore a logo from the University of Brighton, a rival institution. But half the students had their own University of Sussex identity made salient before smelling the shirt, while the other half were randomly selected to have their broader identity as college students made salient.

One might imagine that when it comes to body odor, thinking about oneself specifically as a Sussex student versus a college student in general should have little bearing on how repulsive one finds it. But in fact, students reported less disgust when they smelled a T-shirt from a rival institution if they were thinking about themselves as part of the broader category of students. Making their shared identity salient made the musty shirt a bit more tolerable.

The researchers ran another version of the study in Scotland with students from St. Andrews University.[10] In this case, they had a female student go for a jog in two different T-shirts, one with a navy-blue St. Andrews logo and one with the logo of Dundee, a rival university.

They found that people used more hand sanitizer and spent a longer time washing their hands after holding a stinky shirt associated with the rival university than they did after holding one from their own. A shared sense of social identity again seemed to stop their stomachs from turning (or at least turning as much) when handling the dirty shirts.

Research on smell reveals rather dramatically how identities shape our perception of the world. Whether we're sniffing something pleasing or something nasty, our sensory experiences are shaped by what is inside and what is outside the identity we currently have activated. It is time now to explore more deeply how the lens of identity affects perceptions beyond the boundary—how it affects perceptions of "outsiders."

SEE YOUR FRIENDS CLOSE AND YOUR ENEMIES CLOSER

From the Great Wall of China to the controversial unfinished border wall between Mexico and the United States, humans have invested immense amounts of blood and treasure to keep outsiders at a distance. In some cases, the threats were real, but in others, they were nonexistent or exaggerated.

Over the past few years, some of our research has investigated relationships between group conflict and the experience of space, particularly the perception of physical distance between groups. In one set of studies led by Jenny Xiao, we found that people who felt threatened by an out-group judged that group as physically closer than people who felt more secure did.[11]

People who agreed with statements like "Immigration from Mexico is undermining American culture" thought that Mexico City was closer to their own location than people who did not experience a sense of threat from immigration. We found this pattern when we ran a study with New Yorkers and again when we surveyed people from across the United States. Regardless of where people lived, a sense of threat made the out-group loom closer in their minds.

The out-group also loomed larger. In another study, people who felt this sort of threat thought the volume of immigrants coming across the border into the United States was significantly larger than people who were not threatened did.[12]

Strikingly, this pattern was driven by feelings of what psychologists call symbolic or cultural threats rather than realistic threats. People experiencing symbolic threats feel that their cultures, and therefore their very identities, are being eroded by out-group members. People experiencing realistic threats are focused instead on more practical matters; they may believe, for example, that out-group members are taking their jobs or overusing an important resource. For many Americans, symbolic but not practical concerns about immigration made them exaggerate the proximity of an out-group.

But it is important to note that this was observed only among strongly identified Americans. The people who reported the most pride in their own country were also the ones who had the tightest link between their sense of symbolic threat and their impression that Mexico City was too close for comfort. People who were not deeply identified as Americans did not show the same pattern.

This all changed if people thought there was a strong boundary between the United States and Mexico. After reading that the southern border was "among the most heavily protected in the world," Americans who felt threatened by immigration no longer overestimated their proximity to Mexico City. However, if they were reminded that the border was "frequently crossed" and "largely unsecured," we found a nearly identical pattern to before.

Shortly after we finished this project, Donald Trump ran for president on the promise of building a wall between the United States and Mexico. The idea became such a central part of his campaign that Trump and his supporters would chant "Build that wall! Build that wall!" at his political rallies.[13] Despite the fact that most experts thought a wall was bad policy and ineffective at addressing immigration issues, Trump became obsessed with the wall. He capitalized on the psychology the two of us were seeing in our own studies, exacerbating feelings of symbolic threat to increase supporters' concerns about immigration and immigrants.

Constructing literal and metaphorical barriers to outsiders is a time-tested strategy for gaining political power (one that we will discuss further in chapter 9 when we talk about leadership). But these dynamics don't apply only to immigrants or in political contexts. We found similar patterns of judgments when we examined other forms of social identity.

We started by sending our research team to a baseball game at Yankee Stadium on a beautiful summer night in New York City. As the Yankees fans (along with a mix of tourists and fans of other teams) streamed into the stands, we asked a set of them to fill out questionnaires indicating their favorite team and their feelings toward other teams. Then we handed them unlabeled maps of the East Coast, a five-hundred-mile stretch extending from North Carolina to Maine. We asked each of them to indicate the stadium location of the Yankees' archrivals, the Boston Red Sox (who play at Fenway Park), or of another team in their division, the Baltimore Orioles (who play at Camden Yards). The map included a pin indicating the location of Yankee Stadium, which was roughly halfway between the two other stadiums. Done accurately, the participant would mark an X about 190 miles to the north in the heart of Boston for Fenway Park or about 170 miles to the south in Baltimore for Camden Yards.

It is well known in the baseball world that Yankees and Red Sox fans despise each other. Many consider this the fiercest rivalry in American sports. At the time of our study, the Yankees were leading their division, and the Red Sox were in second place, only one game behind. The Orioles were dead last (a total of twenty-three games behind the Yankees) and had absolutely no hope of making the playoffs. This heated race between the Yankees and the Red Sox was just one more reason for their fans to hate each other after a century of animosity.

Feelings of animosity influenced people's judgments of physical distance. New York Yankees fans thought that the Boston Red Sox stadium was closer than the stadium of the Baltimore Orioles. In reality, it's the other way around. Critically, when we asked the same question of non-Yankees fans at the game, they were more accurate, correctly indicating, on average, that the home of the Orioles was closer to New York than that of the Red Sox.[14]

We also found that it didn't matter if people had been to these cities or felt confident in their judgments. The expertise they might have gained by traveling did not seem to help Yankees fans make more accurate judgments. The intense competition apparently overcame their experience.

These misperceptions had consequences. We ran another study with Yankees fans a year later to see if feelings of proximity to their nemeses might motivate them to engage in discrimination.[15] This time around, we manipulated their sense of closeness by showing them one of two images of the Red Sox and Yankees logos. In one image, the logos were close together (maybe too close for comfort); in the other, they were far away.

Yankees fans who saw the hated Red Sox logo as spatially closer to their own team's were more willing to support discriminatory policies against them. These fans endorsed giving Red Sox fans lower-priority seating at Yankee Stadium. We also showed Yankees fans the stadium's seating chart and had them mark where they thought Red Sox fans should sit. To our surprise, several of these Yankees fans wanted to kick Red Sox fans out of the stadium entirely!

Our studies reveal how social identity can provide a lens for interpreting the world that amplifies intergroup conflict. But we believe this represents only the tip of the iceberg. Aspects of identity can contribute to biases in perception that have enormous repercussions, including starkly negative consequences for justice within legal systems.

VISUAL POLICING

In August 2014, police in St. Louis, Missouri, shot and killed twenty-five-year-old Kajieme Powell, a Black man with a history of mental-health issues. Fewer than twenty seconds elapsed from the time the police arrived on the scene to arrest Mr. Powell for allegedly shoplifting two energy drinks and some doughnuts to the time they fired several bullets at him.

This tragedy unfolded miles from Ferguson, Missouri, where Michael Brown Jr. had been fatally shot by a police officer just days earlier. The violent deaths of these two Black men at the hands of the police launched national protests against police violence.

Police statements about Kajieme Powell's death were not consistent with video evidence. According to the police chief, Mr. Powell had "pulled out a knife and came at the officers, gripping and holding it high" and was "within 2 or 3 feet of the officers" when they shot and killed him.[16] However, a cell phone video of the shooting revealed that Powell was much farther away than a few feet and appeared to have his arms low at his sides.

The killing sparked a fierce debate about what had actually happened and whether the officers' use of force was justified. After a long investigation of forensic, video, and witness evidence, St. Louis circuit attorney Jennifer M. Joyce "determined a criminal violation against either officer could not be proven beyond a reasonable doubt." Her decision not to charge the officers was consistent with a national pattern—very few police officers are charged following deadly interactions with citizens.

When police officers started wearing body cameras, many people thought it would help resolve controversies about what happened during interactions with civilians; the videos would provide an objective account of what actually occurred. The hope was that body-camera footage would hold police and citizens alike accountable. Finally, judgments about what happened during fraught interactions would be grounded in hard evidence. Judges and juries could see with their own eyes what had unfolded in these deadly encounters.

Hundreds of police departments around the world have invested large sums to outfit their officers with body cameras in the hope that it will improve policing. Some departments have randomly assigned officers to wear cameras. Results are mixed and it is not clear that they reduce the amount of force that police use or complaints about police conduct from the public.[17] Another question is whether the videos themselves reduce bias in criminal justice investigations. Do they allow prosecutors, juries, and judges to get a better handle on what actually happened?

Law professor Seth Stoughton of the University of South Carolina created a series of videos to directly investigate how effective body cameras were in creating agreement around police encounters.[18] Stoughton, a former police officer himself, supports initiatives to have officers wear cameras to help determine what happened in these interactions.

Despite Stoughton's hopes, however, people did not see his videos uniformly. Most people usually agreed that the officer in these videos faced a threat to his safety. But people who had a high level of trust in the police were more likely to believe that the officer faced a serious threat to his life than people who distrusted the police were.

As with many real-life encounters caught on tape, the videos were ambiguous, which allowed for people's preconceptions and beliefs about the police to influence their judgments. Like a Rorschach inkblot test, what people saw in these videos tended to be shaped by what they already believed, influencing their interpretations of confrontations between the police and citizens. People differed in their identification with the police and with the civilians in these videos. These affiliations, in turn, guided them to view the same interactions quite differently.

To better understand the role of identification and visual attention during these sorts of judgments, Yael Granot and her colleagues monitored people's eye movements as they watched video clips of physical confrontations between police officers and suspects.[19]

Participants in her studies watched forty-five-second videos of actual altercations between police officers and civilians in which it was ambiguous if the police officers engaged in unethical or violent behavior, such as using too much force when arresting a suspect.

In one clip, an officer attempted to handcuff a suspect who had swallowed a package of drugs and was resisting arrest. They struggled and the officer pushed the suspect against the police cruiser. The suspect then bit the officer's arm, after which the officer hit the suspect on the back of the head. As people watched the videos, the researchers secretly observed their visual attention using an eye-tracker built into the computer monitor. Afterward, the participants were asked if and to what extent the officer should be punished for hitting the suspect.

Despite seeing exactly the same videos, there was a startling lack of agreement among participants. People who identified with the police and spent more time visually focused on the officers in the videos were less likely to want the officers punished than people who did not identify with the police but also had their eyes fixed on what the officers did.

In short, the videos did little to resolve conflicting impressions. Rather, the more attention people paid to the officers, the more polarized they were in their punishment decisions. By directing their attention to the officers, people were able to spin a psychological story about blame that aligned with their preexisting identities.

The fact is that identities provide us with ideas, philosophies, theories, and languages that draw our attention to what matters and help us to explain to ourselves (and others) what is unfolding in the world around us. These identities shape our perception of the social and physical world, altering where we look and how we interpret the environment. This selective attention and filtering process helps explain why people can experience the same events yet come to very different conclusions about what transpired. Thankfully, there are some potential solutions to these challenges.

DIFFERENT PERSPECTIVES

Bias in policing is not the only case where seeing the world through the lens of identity can produce problems for society, but it is one of the most important. Unfortunately, the lens of identity influences not only how third parties judge the actions of police officers but also how police officers judge civilians. To provide just one example, researchers examined nearly one hundred million police stops across the United States from 2011 to 2018 to determine how visual information about racial identity shaped police decisions.[20]

The racial identities of drivers are more visible to police officers during the day; after the sun sets, it is harder to detect the race of someone behind the wheel. This is important because a fair amount of policing involves making decisions in ambiguous circumstances. Is a car being driven erratically? Is a person acting suspicious? Does a driver look like a wanted suspect? How the police handle these little decisions can have big consequences.

If the color of someone's skin affects whether an officer chooses to pull a person over, there should be larger racial disparities in traffic stops during the day than at night, when race is harder to distinguish. This is indeed what the researchers found. Black drivers made up a smaller proportion of traffic stops *after dark* than they did during the day. Under a "veil of darkness," the officers made decisions that were less racially biased. They could no longer use racial identity and stereotypes to make sense of otherwise ambiguous information.

The research team also analyzed police officers' decisions to search a person's car for illegal materials such as drugs or weapons. Here, too, there was evidence of racial bias. At municipal police departments, for example, Black drivers were searched in over 9 percent of traffic stops, Hispanic drivers in 7 percent, and White drivers in only 4 percent.

When searches were conducted, however, officers actually found contraband more often when the driver was White. For these same departments, 18 percent of the White drivers they searched were in possession of illegal materials; this occurred for only 11 percent of Hispanic and 14 percent of Black drivers. So Black drivers were less likely than White drivers to be in possession of illegal materials if they were pulled over, but because they were pulled over significantly more often, Black drivers were arrested more often than White drivers.

These sorts of patterns are due to psychological biases among police officers as they decide every day on the job whom to pull over and whom to search. Their use of visual information—in this case, skin color—shapes how they interpret and act on other information.

It turns out that this is a situation where identity is part of the problem but can also provide a partial solution. A recent large-scale study in Chicago, for example, found that increasing the diversity of police officers made a significant difference in policing behavior.[21] Black and Hispanic officers made fewer stops and arrests and used force less often than White officers. This was especially true in their interactions with Black civilians. When the researchers closely examined the data, they noticed that these differences stemmed from a reduced focus on enforcing low-level offenses among Black civilians. These are the sorts of ambiguous scenarios in which identity-based cues are most likely to guide people's attention and interpretation.

These data show very concretely why representation matters. In the case of policing, hiring more racially and ethnically diverse officers who better represent many of the communities they police can help reduce the aggressive forms of law enforcement that result in racially disparate outcomes. These officers are able to see the world through a different lens, which changes how they interpret and police ambiguous situations.

We believe the same principles apply in other contexts and

organizations. Our identities help us make sense of the world. They reveal many things but obscure others. If we focus on one thing, we inevitably miss something else. Worse, we struggle to recognize our own biases. Though we can readily see how other people's perceptions are fallible, we often fail to see how our own experiences are filtered through the lenses of our identities.

Researchers call this the "bias blind spot," and it is common. One set of studies on 661 Americans found that more than 85 percent believed they were less biased than the average citizen.[22] Remarkably, only a single person acknowledged being *more biased* than average. Understanding that identity shapes our interpretations of everything from sporting events to policing should give us pause. Before we jump to conclusions, it is worth reflecting not only on our potential biases but on the fact that these biases are often invisible to us.

We have focused extensively in this chapter on the ways in which identities shape perception, in part because recognizing biases in ourselves is a step toward a solution. In the next chapter, we will examine how groups shape our very beliefs about the world— and, critically, how we can build identities that strive for accuracy and truth.

CHAPTER 3

SHARING REALITY

One fall day in 1954, readers of the *Chicago Herald* stumbled upon a strange story on the newspaper's back page, an article headlined "Prophecy from Planet Clarion Call to City: Flee That Flood. It'll Swamp Us on Dec. 21, Outer Space Tells Suburbanite." The suburbanite in question was a Mrs. Dorothy Martin, and one of the intrigued readers was Leon Festinger, a social psychologist at the University of Minnesota.

Dorothy Martin was a homemaker living in Chicago. She was also the leader of a local doomsday cult. The newspaper informed its readers that Martin believed she could communicate with superior alien beings—known as the Guardians—from the planets Clarion and Cerus, and that they had given her an urgent and ominous warning. According to Martin, the Guardians had been visiting on flying saucers when they'd noticed disturbing fault lines in the Earth's crust that allowed them to anticipate an imminent and massive flood that would submerge the Western Seaboard of the United States. The aliens, already in close communication with Martin, were kind enough to give her a heads-up, which she had dutifully shared with a local paper.

At the time, Leon Festinger was trying to understand how people dealt with conflicting beliefs; he was puzzled by the fact that people often failed to update their beliefs in the face of logic or counterevidence. Festinger recognized the doomsday prophecy as a perfect opportunity to examine how group dynamics bolster people's convictions.[1]

Festinger and a colleague decided to join the cult—known as the Seekers—to collect data as trusted insiders. They wanted to observe how cult members would react on December 21, the day scheduled for the apocalyptic flood. Festinger knew the prophecy was nonsense. He reasoned that this day would mark the moment when cult members were confronted with irrefutable evidence that their expectations were false. He wanted to be in the room when it happened to see how the Seekers would respond when their entire worldview came crashing down.

By the middle of December, Dorothy Martin announced she had received new and exciting information from the Guardians: She and a loyal group of fellow believers would be rescued from the flood! According to this fortuitous update to the prophecy, they would receive a call at midnight on December 21 and it would provide them with the whereabouts of the spacecraft that would whisk them away to safety. This became a source of hope and a cornerstone belief of the group.

On the evening of December 20, the cult members assembled at Dorothy Martin's house. Only people who could prove they were true believers were allowed in. At the instruction of their leader, they removed all the metal from their bodies, including zippers, bras with underwires, and keys, and waited patiently for their alien escort. It's not hard to imagine how excited the believers must have felt. They were going to meet the aliens for the first time and experience confirmation of their shared reality. It was a big night for the Seekers.

The midnight hour approached. The cult members waited with anticipation.

When the clock finally struck twelve, members of the cult glanced around, curious as to why nothing had happened. Minutes passed. Some looked concerned.

With a sigh of relief, one member noticed that another clock read 11:55 p.m. That must be the correct time. The aliens would make contact in five minutes!

Then that second clock struck midnight.

Nothing.

Seconds ticked by, followed by agonizing minutes. Minutes turned into hours. The impending cataclysm was now mere hours away.

The group sat in stunned silence, confronted with the cold reality that no one was coming for them and, worse, that their entire belief system was wrong. One member began to cry.

Then, just before 5:00 a.m., Mrs. Martin suddenly received another message: "The little group, sitting all night long, has spread so much light that God had saved the world from destruction." They weren't wrong after all! By standing fast and maintaining the faith, the little group of believers had secured salvation for humanity!

The question is, having saved the world, what did they do next? Did they quietly gather up their discarded belongings and retreat back to their families and previous lives? Did they call it a day and move on?

To the contrary, within hours, the Seekers, who had previously shunned interviews, were calling newspapers to broadcast their message of salvation as widely as possible.

Why would the group cling to their belief system even after watching it get debunked? In this chapter, we will explore the lessons that this cult from the 1950s has for our understanding of identity and the nature of belief. Along the way, we'll discuss the important and often very sensible psychological motives that drive people to conform to group norms. Our world is far too complex and confusing for anyone to go it alone, and conforming to our groups' norms is also often how we express our valued identities to the world. This usually works well, but it can produce seriously bad outcomes when groups and organizations become cultlike and are driven by groupthink. Still, groups can adopt accuracy goals and evidence-based identities, both of which help improve the beliefs we share and the decisions we make.

ALL REALITY IS SOCIAL REALITY

An illusion shared by everyone becomes a reality.
—Erich Fromm, *The Dogma of Christ*

At around the same time Festinger was infiltrating the Seekers, social psychologist Solomon Asch was conducting groundbreaking experiments on conformity. In his studies, Asch asked small groups of students at Swarthmore College to complete a series of exceedingly easy visual tasks.[2] On each trial, the students were presented with a set of three vertical lines and asked to identify which one was the same length as a fourth line. A toddler could do it. (We know this because we gave this test to our own children when they were toddlers!)

When participants completed the task on their own, they almost always gave the right answers. But Asch wanted to see what people would do if they were in a group, so he had the students sit around a table and announce their answers when the experimenter held up the simple visual stimuli. What participants didn't realize, however, was that there was actually only one real participant in each session; all the other members of the group were Asch's stooges, who had been instructed to answer the questions incorrectly at critical points during the experiment. The situation was also arranged so that the unsuspecting real participant always responded last.

Thus, on those occasions when all the other students gave an incorrect answer, the real participant was presented with a choice: Should he report the obviously correct answer or conform to the group and give the wrong answer? As Chico Marx says in the movie *Duck Soup,* "Who are you gonna believe, me or your own eyes?"

Seventy-six percent of Solomon Asch's participants who were confronted with obvious discrepancies between the visual evidence and other people's erroneous responses did in fact ignore their own eyes and echo the incorrect answer at least once. On average, people conformed about a third of the time. Fewer than one in four participants completely resisted the power of the group on every trial.

Why would they do this? Why would people conform and give answers they must have known were false? If you're thinking, *Peer pressure,* you're right. Peer pressure—which psychologists call *normative influence*—plays a key role in producing *conformity.* And we know that this was a factor in Asch's experiments because when he gave participants the chance to respond anonymously, writing their answers down instead of saying them aloud, the number of incorrect answers was reduced to near zero.

This type of conformity pressure is usually driven by a person's desire to fit in and avoid the social discomfort and potential ostracism that often come from deviance. But this is not the only reason that people conform. We have run similar experiments in which people were given a somewhat more difficult visual task, one that required them to decide whether two shapes in different orientations were the same or different. In this case, the answer wasn't always immediately clear. After they looked at the shapes for a few seconds, we presented them with a pie chart that supposedly showed the proportions of prior participants who had given each answer.

Our participants gave significantly more correct answers when they saw a pie chart where the majority was correct and significantly more incorrect answers when the majority on the pie chart was incorrect. But here's the thing: All of our participants were doing this alone on computers in small cubicles, where no one else could possibly observe their responses. Rather than conforming to fit in, they were using the pie charts showing what other people had done as a source of information to guide their own responses. This type of *conformity* is known as *informational influence,* and it is motivated by a desire to get things right based on the assumption that other people are generally a good source of information.[3] When people are not sure how to act, they look to others for clues about what to think and how to behave.

Informational influence was not a factor in the original Asch studies because the task in question was so simple that people had no need to rely on others for information. But when tasks or situations are more difficult or ambiguous, as they so often are in life, we turn to other people to help us figure out what is going on. Adults often try to discourage teenagers from conforming to peer pressure with admonishments like "Just say no!," but in many cases, conforming to the behavior of others is a perfectly sensible thing for them to do.

If you assume that other people are roughly as well informed as you are, it is rational to give their preferences equal weight as your own when you make a decision.[4] Imagine, for example, that you are trying to choose between two audiobooks before setting off on a long road trip alone. You have a mild preference for one of the books, but you know that a good friend of yours recently chose to listen to the other one (although you do not know what she thought of it after listening). In this situation, assuming that your friend has about as much knowledge and expertise as you, it is rational to essentially flip a mental coin and opt for whichever choice randomly comes up. In other words, you have as much reason to go with your friend's preference as yours. Maybe your friend knows something that you do not.

Next, imagine that two of your close friends have chosen the other audiobook. Now it is two to one in favor of that choice, and you don't even need to flip a coin; you should opt for their preference instead of your own. This type of dynamic may contribute to the development of behavioral "cascades"—otherwise known as fads—in which preferences for particular musicians, books, clothing styles, haircuts, college majors, or verbal expressions spread rapidly through large populations. If you look through old magazines, you can see countless trends, like shoulder pads and bell-bottom jeans, that were fashionable for a while and then disappeared, though probably not forever. Assuming that other people have insight into what sounds good, looks good, et cetera, we are often quick to follow the crowd no matter what our initial opinions or impressions were.

This idea might help to explain why fads and fashions often end very quickly as people shift their preferences to something new.[5] As a cascade grows, you can assume that more and more people are basing their decisions on what other people are doing and not on their own knowledge and expertise. At some point, it becomes clear that what other people are doing is not about what tastes good or looks good but merely about what is popular.

Now, divergent and different choices made by smaller numbers of people become more informative because presumably they had a good reason for making those more unusual decisions. Suddenly today's fashion starts to appear faded and tired, and you're ready to join the crowd for the next big thing!

So we go along with others when we want to fit in and also when we think they are good sources of information. A third and related reason we conform is to *express valued identities*.[6] As discussed in chapter 1, the groups we belong to have norms that articulate "how we do things around here"—the patterns of thought, feeling, and action that define what it means to be a member of a particular group. The more we identify with a group, the more we tend to want to exemplify its norms in our own behavior.

People sometimes describe conformity as "contagious," implying that ideas and behaviors spread virally across entire populations, even the whole species. But contagion is not the best metaphor because, unlike most viruses, conformity typically stops at the group's edge. It is bounded, such that we are much more likely to conform to in-group norms than the norms of out-groups. All three motives for conformity contribute to this. We care more about being accepted by fellow in-group members and fitting in with them. We often assume that our own groups are smarter and wiser than others and thus are better sources of information. And it is our own groups' identities that we want to express.

Indeed, conformity is not just bounded by group borders; it can even become oppositional, as when one group of people opts not to do something simply because another group is doing it, or vice versa.[7] This often happens when wealthy or hip groups adopt different styles once a trend they had embraced reaches the masses. It is easy to see how these sorts of identity dynamics can be problematic in highly polarized environments if defiance drives some groups to embrace less accurate beliefs or engage in self-destructive behaviors so they can maintain distinctiveness from rivals. You can sometimes see this dynamic on social media when people post videos of themselves burning their shoes or destroying their coffeemakers to signal that they reject a particular company's political stance.

But although it has a dark side, conformity serves critical functions in human groups. The capacity of our species to share ideas and information and thereby coordinate behavior is what sets humans apart from other species, including other primates. As cognitive scientists Philip Fernbach and Steve Sloman pointed out, "Chimpanzees can surpass young children on numerical and spatial reasoning tasks, but they cannot come close on tasks that require collaborating with another individual to achieve a goal. Each of us knows only a little bit, but together we can achieve remarkable feats."[8]

No single mind can master and retain all the information needed to successfully navigate the world. Knowledge isn't so much what's in our heads—it's what is shared between us. When Isaac Newton wrote, "If I have seen further it is by standing on the shoulders of Giants," he was expressing his gratitude for the collective nature of knowledge.[9]

Left alone, humans are not well equipped to separate fact from fiction. If you scoffed at the notion that an alien spaceship was coming to rescue the Seekers, that is probably because you belong to communities skeptical about UFO encounters and end-of-the-world narratives. It is not that you lack a social identity—it is that your beliefs are aligned with those of entirely different groups of people.

Although relying on one's communities is normally much better than going it alone, there are obviously some important exceptions. When people are overly influenced by charlatans, cult leaders, or propagandists, they can be led terribly astray. We might be tempted to think that cult members are a special breed, but a similar form of group psychology can afflict people in any area of life, including politics and the corporate world. We do not have to go so far as an actual cult to see what happens when groups ramp up pressure on their members to conform, grow insular in the information they seek, and come to believe too strongly their own stories about themselves and their place in the world. If these dynamics are left unchecked, the economic and human costs can be profound.

AS SOLID AS MANHATTAN

Early one morning in May of 2019, Dom roused his grumbling kids from bed, handed them each a granola bar, and loaded them into the car. There was little traffic at six thirty on a Sunday and in minutes they arrived at their destination: the top deck of Lehigh University's Alumni Memorial parking garage. There they joined a surprisingly large assembly of people, many still pajama-clad, almost all of them clutching coffee. Despite the early hour and the austere location, the crowd had an air of sleepy festivity. They were there to watch Martin Tower fall.

Martin Tower was the tallest building ever constructed in Pennsylvania's Lehigh Valley. Erected in the early 1970s, this imposing structure served as headquarters for the Bethlehem Steel

Corporation, at one time the second-largest steel producer in the United States. The company was integral to the nation's military might, supplying materials for more than a thousand ships during World War II. Steel from Bethlehem built the Golden Gate Bridge, and in 1955 Bethlehem Steel ranked number eight on the list of Fortune 500 companies.[10]

Martin Tower was intentionally built as a symbol of the company's strength. Unintentionally, however, it also symbolized aspects of the insular and hubristic corporate culture that, in the long run, contributed to its demise. The tower was constructed in the shape of a plus sign, not for any structural reason but to appease the egos of managers and executives by maximizing the number of corner offices.

If you were in management, Bethlehem Steel was a good company to work for. Dining with executives was famously a "four-star" experience; long lunches were taken in an elegantly appointed room replete with silver tableware. At the time, many industries did important business over rounds of golf, and Bethlehem Steel actually built golf courses for their managers near many of their plants.

At one point, nine of the twelve highest-paid executives in all of America worked for Bethlehem Steel. They had every reason to be satisfied with themselves, and they felt that their position was impregnable. As CEO Eugene Grace noted, the dramatic skyline soaring from the granite of nearby Manhattan Island, much of it built with Bethlehem's steel, was emblematic of the solidity of the company.

But out there in the real world, all was not well. Foreign competition and technological changes were on the rise. These forces accelerated during the second half of the twentieth century, ultimately posing a mortal challenge to the entire American steel industry. Some companies were able to adapt to new external realities and survive, but Bethlehem Steel was not.

There are, of course, many factors that contribute to the demise of a major corporation, but the Bethlehem Steel story is a cautionary tale about what can happen when an organization becomes insular—seeking information only from inside and getting caught up in its own mythology.

The corporation had only four CEOs for the first sixty-six years of its existence. Eugene Grace served into his eighties; in his later years, he sometimes fell asleep in board meetings, so everyone would wait for him to wake up before carrying on. The board itself was composed mostly of company insiders, as were the managers, who were generally promoted internally rather than recruited from experienced and increasingly dangerous competitors. In an industry that became hypercompetitive, the lack of outsider perspectives may well have been fatal.

In the end, what finally killed Bethlehem Steel were the costs associated with pensions and health benefits put into place when the company was thriving and the bottom line was strong.[11] The management spent lavishly on perks and benefits while failing to look ahead. They mistakenly assumed that tomorrow would be like today and deferred all of these costs to the future. But when the future arrived, the problems were too big to fix. In 2001 the company went bankrupt, and by 2003 it had been dissolved.

And so, shortly after seven o'clock on a clear morning in 2019, the crowd atop the parking garage saw flickers of light run down the sides of the plus-sign-shaped building as explosive charges took out its structural supports. As the spectators held their breath, Martin Tower held steady for just a moment before collapsing in on itself in a massive cloud of dust.

CORPORATE CULTS

We started this chapter with the story of a cult. Bethlehem Steel was by no means a cult, but as an organization it exhibited some

71

of the same pathologies of belief—in their own superiority, wisdom, and resilience—that characterize groups on a cultlike continuum. As Bethlehem Steel declined in the late twentieth century, another major American company was moving even further along that trajectory.

In the mid-1980s, Kenneth Lay took the helm of a new company, Enron, the product of a merger between two energy behemoths. Over the next decade, guided by Lay and a tight-knit group of senior leaders, Enron was transformed from a traditional energy company grounded in oil and gas infrastructure—physical assets—to a financial organization engaged in massive commodities trading.[12] The company was wildly successful; in the year 2000, it employed more than twenty thousand people and claimed revenues of over a hundred billion dollars—at least on paper.

As it turned out, however, much of Enron's apparent value was illusory, built on dodgy accounting practices rather than real profits. The fraud was multifaceted, complex, and creative. For example, executives managed to keep significant debts off Enron's books by transferring them to limited partnerships that they then treated as separate companies. When this practice was eventually challenged by their auditors, the house of cards began to collapse.

The scale of the fraud at Enron was too vast to attribute to just a "few bad apples," although former president George Bush did just that. Commentators, including writers at the *Economist* magazine, suggested that Enron should be understood as "some sort of evangelical cult." Organizational researchers Dennis Tourish and Naheed Vatcha have subjected this idea to serious scrutiny and concluded that the analogy is apt. In particular, they note that cults have a variety of features exhibited by Enron in its heyday.[13]

For example, cults usually have charismatic leaders. For the Seekers, it was Dorothy Martin, allegedly blessed with special powers to communicate with higher beings. At Enron, senior leadership was held in almost mythic esteem. The executives considered themselves and were widely perceived to be genius revolutionaries, upending a staid and conservative industry in pursuit of vastly larger profits.

Jeffrey Skilling, who succeeded Kenneth Lay as CEO, embraced a characterization of himself as Darth Vader, a reputation he earned because he was "a master of the energy universe who had the ability to control people's minds. He was at the peak of his strength, and he intimidated everyone."[14] He referred to his traders as Storm Troopers.

Cult leaders promulgate "totalistic visions" for their groups, transcendent ideologies that explain everything and provide clear guides to action. There is no vision more encompassing, for example, than one that claims the world is about to end and there is but one means of securing salvation. But at Enron, the vision was of the company becoming much more than just a major player in the energy industry.

As a massive banner overhanging the building's entrance said, Enron's mission was to transform FROM THE WORLD'S LEADING ENERGY COMPANY—TO THE WORLD'S LEADING COMPANY. Tourish and Vatcha note that although this was a secular rather than religious or apocalyptic vision, "it promised people heaven on earth. If the company were to achieve its goals, unimagined wealth and happiness would be the lot of those fortunate enough to be employees at the time."

As with cults generally, Enron used its recruitment procedures as a way to indoctrinate employees right from the start. The selection process was notoriously intense and competitive, involving at one point a rapid-fire interrogation with eight different interviewers. Anyone who made it through the gauntlet and got a job would feel that he or she had been specially selected to join an elite crew. These new employees' sense of specialness was reinforced and tied to their identity with the company; "Enronians were frequently told, and came to believe, that they were the brightest and best employees in the world." This praise was matched by generous compensation and

THE POWER OF US

large bonuses for people who were deemed sufficiently aggressive at pursuing the company's interests.

Finally, in order to maintain the faith, Enron's leadership brooked no dissent. Among other measures, they employed a harsh evaluation system known as "rank and yank," which created a highly competitive environment and enabled managers to quickly get rid of anyone they did not like. As other writers on Enron have noted, "In the process of trying to quickly and efficiently separate from the company those employees who were not carrying their weight, Enron created an environment where most employees were afraid to express their opinions or to question unethical and potentially illegal business practices. Because the rank-and-yank system was both arbitrary and subjective, it was easily used by managers to reward blind loyalty and quash brewing dissent."[15]

These cultlike features—highly charismatic leaders, a totalistic vision, careful indoctrination, and elimination of dissent—create groups and organizations with highly enthusiastic followers. Deeply devoted to the mission and insulated from divergent perspectives, they become blind to the group's internal inconsistencies, exacting costs, and even potential illegality. And this worldview is socially reinforced by fellow group members—just like the Seekers in Dorothy Martin's apocalyptic cult.

When its illusions and false beliefs came crashing down, Enron went bankrupt and disappeared. Kenneth Lay and Jeffrey Skilling were tried together and convicted of fraud; Lay died before his sentencing, but Skilling was sent to prison. Other executives also went to jail. Thousands of employees lost their jobs and their pensions. The dream was over. And in this regard, what happens to members of a corporate cult differs from what often happens to members of a group like the Seekers when their expectations do not come to pass.

WHEN PROPHECIES FAIL

Fifty years after Dorothy Martin's extraterrestrial friends failed to materialize, a preacher named Harold Camping made another doomsday prophecy. Camping, president of a Christian broadcasting network called Family Radio, predicted that the Rapture would occur on May 21, 2011.

Mr. Camping devoted countless hours of his radio program to talking about Judgment Day and spent millions of dollars on billboards to warn people in more than forty countries. This publicity was successful, and his prophecy attracted the attention of many prominent news outlets, including the *New York Times,* the Associated Press, and *Time* magazine.

It also attracted the attention of a team of economists who decided to build on Festinger's original study of the Seekers. Being economists, they wanted to measure the power of belief in real dollars. And they added a crucial control group that had been missing from the investigation of the Seekers. The economists included a set of Seventh-Day Adventists who were somewhat similar to Camping's followers in that many of them did expect the Rapture to occur during their lifetimes but who did not believe, despite Camping's prophecy, that it would occur on May 21. This allowed the researchers to directly compare the reactions of two similar religious groups with divergent apocalyptic beliefs.

The researchers approached Family Radio followers and Seventh-Day Adventists outside of Bible-study classes and offered them money. But they had to make a choice—they could have five dollars right away or up to five hundred dollars (the amounts varied) four weeks later.[16] Critically, however, participants would not receive the larger sum until after May 21, the date scheduled for doomsday.

Any rational investor reading this will realize that waiting just a few weeks for a larger sum of money gives you a rate of return better than any fund in the stock market. But of course, that only matters if you think the world will exist long enough for you to get the payoff!

The Seventh-Day Adventists acted like people in previous economic studies. On average, they were willing to wait to receive the money if they could get at least seven dollars in the near future rather than five dollars immediately. The most that anyone in the control group required to wait for a few weeks was twenty dollars. They were willing to be patient to earn a few extra bucks. A wise financial choice.

In contrast, and to a person, Harold Camping's followers wanted the money now. They would consider delaying the five-dollar payoff only for a very high price. Indeed, the vast majority turned down the chance to get several hundred dollars in a few weeks, insisting on being paid immediately.

So what actually happened on May 21, 2011?

While the members of the research team weren't embedded in the cult like Festinger's team was, they had the next best vantage point: they were able to watch the group's message board on Yahoo. In the days before the predicted Rapture—which, according to Camping, would begin in the first time zone to experience sunset on May 21 and travel around the world from there—the board mainly contained messages of faith and hope. The board went silent a few hours before the first time zone's sunset.

Then, as the moment of the prophecy came and went, activity began to pick up again. The posts revealed the same sorts of reactions that Festinger had observed half a century earlier. Rather than abandoning hope, followers cast about for some sort of explanation that would allow them to maintain the central tenets of the prophecy. People proposed alternative future times for the Rapture, and as each new prediction failed to deliver, a revision was quickly suggested.

This continued until Mr. Camping made his own announcement on May 23. In a new revelation, he said that although the Rapture had not been detectable in the physical realm, a "spiritual judgment" had indeed occurred, initiating the beginning of the end of the world. Despite the apparent contradictory evidence, he and his followers were not wrong, and things were still on track. It is hard to imagine a more perfect replication of the Seekers in the age of the internet.

Why do cult members respond this way when prophecies fail?

Having observed the Seekers, Leon Festinger and his colleagues proposed that when people's identities and beliefs are seriously called into question, it produces immense feelings of discomfort—a state known as *cognitive dissonance*. It might seem rational for people to simply abandon the group, return to their family and friends, and try to make a fresh start. But people will go to incredible lengths to preserve their identity and the group's shared sense of reality. For deeply committed members, it is often easier to ignore contradictions or search for new information that helps reduce feelings of dissonance.

Most of us have other identities and social connections we can turn to when an aspect of our lives hits a major snag. When things are going poorly at the office, you can seek solace at the end of the day by being with your family, by logging into social media to connect with friends, or by turning on the TV to cheer on your favorite team. These alternate identities provide a psychological buffer when something goes wrong. But the Seekers, Family Radio followers, and possibly many Enron employees were in too deep. This created an enormous incentive for them to rationalize or justify events in ways that bolstered their identities and their groups.

The key to maintaining beliefs in the face of countervailing evidence is social support. Isolated believers can rarely withstand overwhelming evidence such as that provided by the failure of a prophecy. Indeed, the importance of social support in maintaining a sense of shared reality may cause people—as we saw with the Seekers—not only to revise their beliefs when they are challenged by reality but also to proselytize in an attempt to grow the number of believers. As Festinger wrote, "If more and more people can be persuaded that the system of belief is correct, then clearly it must, after all, be correct."[17]

This pattern of doubling down on beliefs is a common occurrence when group prophecies fail. Examining how religious groups throughout history have reacted when their predictions are unfulfilled, Festinger observed that "in spite of the failure of the prophecy, the fires of fanaticism increased...the failure seemed to excite even greater exhibitions of loyalty."

As we write this, we see a similar dynamic playing out among followers of the QAnon conspiracy theory, whose predictions about the 2020 presidential election in the United States have been disconfirmed repeatedly. People often think that conspiracy theorists are fundamentally different from others. But we have found that many conspiracy theorists are attracted to these sorts of belief systems because of identity goals. They are attached to conspiratorial beliefs that align with their identities and gain a sense of belonging from sharing those beliefs with fellow adherents.[18]

AVOIDING GROUPTHINK

We certainly aren't claiming that groups are inevitably or invariably cultlike. But the dynamics of identity that drive people to seek shared realities even in the face of contradictory information do affect groups of all sorts. A related scientific literature has famously described these dynamics as *groupthink*.

According to Irving Janis, originator of the idea, a clear case of groupthink occurred a year into John F. Kennedy's presidency when his administration launched a land invasion of Cuba on a remote area of the island known as the Bay of Pigs.[19] The goal was to overthrow Cuban leader Fidel Castro, a Communist and perennial thorn in the side of American economic and foreign policy interests.

Planning for the secret military operation had begun during the administration of JFK's predecessor, Dwight D. Eisenhower. To avoid involving U.S. troops, the CIA had trained fourteen hundred Cuban exiles, preparing them to storm the Bahía de Cochinos and march to Havana. The expatriates were eager to return home and topple a leader they regarded as dictatorial and illegitimate. American thinking was that this would inspire the Cuban people to rise up against Castro, striking a powerful blow against Communist ideology.

Instead, the Cuban exiles were met and quickly overwhelmed by twenty thousand Cuban soldiers. Within four days, more than sixty had been killed and over eleven hundred captured. U.S. ships attempted to evacuate some of the remaining fighters but were ultimately forced to retreat under Cuban fire. The Bay of Pigs invasion was a disaster and a humiliation for Kennedy's still-young presidency.

Kennedy later asked, "How could we have been so stupid?"

Regrettably, even the smartest people can make stupid decisions. It might be easy to dismiss the behavior of some cults. But the Kennedy administration—like Enron—was loaded with brilliant people. Unfortunately, individual intelligence is hardly a cure for social stupidity. Research has found that a person's tendency to approach problems in ways that are likely to confirm what he or she already believes is unrelated to cognitive ability.[20] And group dynamics may exacerbate the problem.

Irving Janis argued that these very smart people had fallen victim to groupthink. Groupthink occurs when a group of people arrive at irrational decisions out of a desire for social conformity. This can be especially powerful when time is an issue and people have to express opinions and objections publicly and to group members who are higher in status. Pressure to maintain harmony and cohesion in these circumstances can lead people to agree at all costs, even when many may privately harbor serious doubts about a decision. Groupthink gives the illusion of a shared reality when none actually exists.

Analyzing the Bay of Pigs decision-making, Janis found that Kennedy's advisers had reason to think the invasion would fail but refrained from expressing their reservations out of concern for seeming "soft" or "un-daring." No one spoke out against it. Yet, as one of Kennedy's advisers later said, "Had one senior advisor opposed the adventure, I believe that Kennedy would have canceled it."

The groupthink idea has inspired decision-makers to take steps to avoid these traps. Leaders are advised to let their subordinates speak before they express their own views. They may appoint people to serve as designated devil's advocates, charged with challenging the group's consensus regardless of their own opinions. One approach that we, as researchers, are very familiar with involves a type of independent-review process.

Imagine what would have happened if Kennedy had sent Eisenhower's plan to his senior advisers and asked them each to write an anonymous critique. He likely would have received a scattershot of perspectives rather than uniform agreement. Kennedy could then have reviewed their opinions and reached his own informed, but independent, decision about how to proceed. No one would have needed to speak out publicly, and the president could have digested his advisers' thoughts and possible objections before expressing his own preferences.

We cannot know how the Bay of Pigs invasion might have turned out with a different, more rigorous advice-seeking process. But we do know that peer review helps root out biased decision-making among scholars and scientists. Every time a scientific paper is submitted to a journal for publication, it goes through this type of scrutiny. In most cases, the paper is sent to an editor who then sends it to a handful of anonymous reviewers who are experts in the field. They are tasked with finding all of the errors, holes in logic, and unsatisfactory conclusions that they can. Many times the process is double-blinded, meaning that the reviewers do not know who the authors are and the authors will never know who the reviewers are.

For most researchers, this process usually results in a rejection. But if their work is deemed sufficiently rigorous and robust, they are invited to make extensive revisions and then resubmit the paper for another round of review. And research suggests that even papers that are initially rejected tend to get better when they are submitted to another journal. This admittedly painful process is how researchers produce scientific advances and expert knowledge. And it does not end there. Once a paper is published, other scientists often weigh in with their own critiques or attempt to replicate findings in their own labs. Each finding and theory is understood to be provisional, and knowledge increases slowly and painstakingly over time.

Peer review is not perfect, but it provides a remarkable antidote to groupthink. Receiving reviews from scientists who disagree about the strengths and weaknesses of your paper can be annoying (trust us, we get irritated too!). Harnessing a diversity of opinions can also slow down the publication process. But when you get a vaccination, fly in a plane, or turn on your computer, you can thank the peer-review process for improving the scientific foundations behind modern medicine and technology.

EVIDENCE-BASED IDENTITIES

In the traditional formulation of groupthink, a group's goal of accuracy is pitted against goals of consensus and cohesion. But when archives related to the Bay of Pigs disaster were opened up, some of the players involved published memoirs, and more materials became available, psychologist Roderick Kramer reevaluated the groupthink explanation.[21] Reviewing a much broader array of evidence than

Irving Janis had, he concluded that the problem with the Kennedy administration's decision-making was not necessarily that people were suppressing views that would have increased the chances of military success but that they were not really thinking about it in those terms to begin with.

Kramer argued that rather than focusing on how to maximize the chances of operational success, Kennedy and his advisers focused on making choices that would play well politically for the administration or at least minimize the domestic political fallout. He suggested that rather than calling their decision-making a product of groupthink, it could be better thought of as the result of "politicothink."

This highlights an important point: groups can have different types of goals and may develop patterns or norms for the sorts of goals that drive their decision-making. And as norms, these patterns tend to be reinforced and enforced. For example, if the two of us were to start sharing dubious news stories on social media, not only would we find our in-boxes full of corrections from our friends, but it would raise more than a few eyebrows in our scientific community. Some of our professional opportunities would probably dry up, we would get fewer invitations to give talks, and we might slowly be removed from important committees.

This is not to say that either of us is perfect! When we do share misinformation or make a less than robust claim, our colleagues are quick to point it out. If we make errors in this book, we have little doubt that our colleagues will let us know—perhaps with a polite note or possibly with a damning critique on Twitter or in a science blog. If we do not acknowledge our errors, we will surely suffer even more in the eyes of our community. These informal sanctions operate because our identity as scientists comes with strong expectations that we will use empirical analysis to arrive at verifiable conclusions. The norm of pursuing accuracy is one that this identity holds very dear, and it is a critical part of the way that each generation of scientists is socialized.

Of course, the socialization process is somewhat different for each scientist and is influenced by the values and actions of mentors and immediate peers. But for many of us, when we see colleagues defending a debunked theory or dismissing a string of failed replications of their work, it casts doubt on their identity as good scientists. The expectation is that they should update their thinking or conduct more research to reconcile the differences between their conclusions and those of their critics. Scientists who do this tend to rise in others' esteem, while those who cling to theories in spite of contradictory evidence tend to drop in stature.

Scientists are far from alone in valuing evidence-based reasoning; investigative journalists, lawyers, judges, investors, engineers, and many others are constantly evaluated in terms of their capacity to rigorously interrogate reality. If they were not, people would not rely on the news, hire expensive lawyers, put money in mutual funds, or drive across bridges without a thought to their structural integrity. When these folks fail to draw sound conclusions, they correct their mistakes as quickly as possible or risk losing clients and finding themselves unemployed. All of these professions thrive when they use editorial, legal, or technical professional standards that enforce rigor. It is not because these fields are populated by perfect people; rather, their strength lies in the values and the institutions that sustain these norms of accuracy.

Above, we suggested that independent peer-review-type processes can provide an antidote to conformist decision-making. But peer reviewers, of course, are also flawed. There is a worry that the biases of reviewers, especially if they are widely held or systemic, could negatively affect the whole enterprise.

We recently analyzed the value of the peer-review process for rooting out political bias within our own community of psychological researchers. According to several surveys, the vast majority of social scientists self-categorize as liberal in their political beliefs.[22] In fact, one survey of social psychologists found that over 89 percent of the field self-identified as liberal; less than 3 percent identified as conservative.[23]

This imbalance led conservative political commentator Arthur Brooks to propose that unconscious partisan bias might be undercutting the quality of research. He quoted one scientist as saying, "Expecting trustworthy results on politically charged topics from an ideologically incestuous community is downright delusional." Brooks noted that even scrupulous researchers could be affected by bias, and he suggested, in particular, that commonly held ideas that align with liberal values may receive a lower standard of scrutiny.

Of course, this is a distinct possibility. If partisan identities are guiding research, it seems quite plausible that some form of bias or groupthink might be taking place in the scientific review process. In fact, we ran an informal poll, to which 699 of our peers on Twitter responded, asking colleagues whether they expected liberal or conservative findings to be less likely to replicate. Forty-three percent thought liberal findings would be less likely to replicate, whereas only 13 percent thought that conservative findings would be less likely to replicate (the other 44 percent expected to find no difference). In other words, many people shared the concern that liberal bias might be leaking into the research literature, making it a shaky foundation to build on.

Yet we suspected that peer review and the critical norms associated with a scientific identity might help root out this problem.[24] To test this, Diego Reinero and other members of Jay's lab analyzed 218 psychology experiments that included over a million participants.[25] Each of these studies had later been replicated by another lab. Comparing the original results to their replications, we wanted to see if the results held up better or worse depending on whether their conclusions were aligned with the partisan political preferences of the field. If liberal scientists were engaging in groupthink or politicothink, we would expect that they might submit flimsier studies aligned with their political identities and also maybe go a little easier on similar studies as reviewers. This would eventually create a body of published research rife with political bias.

After we gathered this stack of academic papers, we took steps to check our own biases. We recruited graduate students from across the political spectrum to read a short summary of each paper. We asked the students to determine whether the findings in each paper supported a liberal worldview, a conservative worldview, or something in between.

We wrote down our analysis plans in a time-stamped online document before we analyzed the data. This prevented us from doing anything to misrepresent our results—it is a strategy to check our own biases (even if they are unconscious). We also teamed up with a researcher who had very different predictions from our team to see if he would come up with the same results using his own preferred approach. Jay warned his lab, "Someone is going to hate us no matter how these results turn out."

Then we crunched the numbers.

The results surprised us in a number of ways. First of all, very few studies were seen as politically slanted. Despite the fact that the field is highly populated by liberals, very few of the studies aligned clearly with those beliefs. Even our most conservative raters failed to see much of a liberal slant in the literature.

Next, we examined whether more liberal findings were less robust than conservative findings. This was our big research question. If liberal groupthink was taking place, the more liberal findings should also be more flimsy and less likely to replicate. However, if anonymous peer review was working as planned, there should be little or no difference in the replicability of liberal or conservative findings. Weaknesses in logic and data should be rooted out by reviewers and editors judging the work through the lens of their scientific rather than political identities.

The good news is that we found no difference in the replication rates of liberal or conservative findings. Liberal and conservatively oriented studies were also similar on other measures of research quality, like the strength of their findings (known as the "effect size") and the quality of their methods.

There was no trace of liberal groupthink. It seems that psychological scientists were, for the most part, able to put their politics aside when they conducted and reviewed research. Instead of exhibiting rank partisanship, they were largely able to channel the values and norms of their scientific identity. This should give outsiders—and researchers—greater reason to trust the data; the institutions scientists have built seem to be fairly immune to the patterns of thought that can afflict political administrations and other types of groups.

Other studies have found similar patterns. One analyzed whether the abstracts of academic conference presentations were biased in favor of liberals. Admittedly, these conference presentations did not undergo the normal scrutiny of peer review at a journal. Again, experts predicted that there would be clear evidence of liberal bias. The authors did find modest evidence of liberal bias in this case. For example, abstracts were slightly more likely to mention conservatives as the target of study than liberals. But the evidence of bias was much weaker than predicted; the experts expected to find far more than they actually observed.[26]

This is good news for society because it underscores the integrity of the scientific process. But it also offers a lesson for people outside of science: there are norms and institutional practices that can be used to promote accuracy even in the face of strong political beliefs. This may seem hard to believe—even the scientists themselves expected to see more bias. But if we were hired by a company to root out groupthink, we would likely come up with a solution that looks a lot like the peer-review process. If Bethlehem Steel and Enron had had mechanisms for input and oversight from independent, anonymous experts, would they have sustained such cultish and ultimately self-destructive cultures? Peer review is far from perfect, but it appears quite useful for addressing this particular problem of group behavior.

Scientists continue to revise and improve our peer-review procedures. Many journals now make research plans, materials, data, and analysis code fully available during peer review. Some journals have created badges—just like Boy Scouts and Girl Scouts—to signal when people are using best practices. We have also created new systems for sharing work and getting feedback before and after peer review, with the understanding that even published papers deserve ongoing scrutiny. Just as important, we continue to analyze and evaluate these innovations as new data roll in. In fact, there is an entire field dedicated to studying the behavior of scientists, called meta-science.

Commitment to accuracy as a central goal is hardly specific to science. By valuing smart criticism, groups and organizations can help foster dissent and improve decision-making. Unfortunately, many leaders act like John F. Kennedy during the planning of the Bay of Pigs. They are the first to share their opinions at meetings, signaling what they value and discouraging dissent. They crush, perhaps unintentionally, the sorts of questions and comments that can identify problems or lead to creative new ideas. This might seem strategically useful for making quick decisions, but it can exact enormous costs in the long run.

ACCURACY IN A DIVIDED WORLD

By this point we hope we have convinced you that humans' understanding of the world is shaped by other humans—that our realities are fundamentally social. Yet, although this is true, people still tend to believe—most of the time, anyway—that they see the world objectively. This phenomenon is known to psychologists as *naive realism*, because people naively assume that they see reality for what it is.

As a result of naive realism, when other people disagree with you, especially if they are members of other groups, you often dismiss them as uninformed, irrational, or biased.

Whereas people tend to think that their own groups see reality more or less for what it is—that they have a good handle on things—they often perceive out-groups as deluded, conformist, and generally incompetent. To illustrate this point, a clever study conducted by researchers at the University of Queensland asked one set of people to name an animal that they felt captured the essence of an in-group they were proud to belong to; they asked another set to name an animal they felt best represented an out-group they would not want to be associated with.[27] Participants in the first group listed noble animals like lions, wolves, tigers, and dolphins. Participants in the second one, however, nominated species known for blind conformity or nefarious intent: sheep and lemmings, snakes and hyenas.

These sorts of assumptions can make it difficult to resolve disagreements of fact between groups. If you enter a discussion assuming that the people on the other side are a bunch of idiots or ideologues, you are not going to win many new friends. Nor is your mind going to be opened to the possibility that you might be wrong.

This particular aspect of identity and group psychology poses a significant problem to society, amplified in our time by political divisions and social media. When groups cannot agree on basic facts, it erodes the foundations for compromise and provides a basis for intractable intergroup conflict. In the age of the internet, it feels easier than ever for people to form their own cultlike cocoons.

Consider debates about vaccination. If one group believes vaccinations are the key to preventing diseases like polio, measles, and COVID-19, and another group thinks that vaccines contain toxins that cause autism and are part of a conspiracy to control people, there is little ground for compromise. Scientists are unlikely to believe the conspiracy theories, and anti-vaxxers are unconvinced by yet another study debunking the link between autism and vaccines. This can lead both sides to retreat from the conversation and spend more time with like-minded others.[28]

People choose doctors, school districts, friends, and jobs that align with their identities. It is easier to avoid conflict and find people who provide a feeling of affirmation than face the discomfort of engaging with people who do not agree with you.

Societies around the world are now grappling with how to stop, or at least slow, the viral spread of misinformation and disinformation online. Social media companies like Facebook and Twitter are experimenting with attaching fact-checks and disclaimers ("This is a disputed claim") to contested and factually dubious messages. They are also increasingly taking steps to remove users and accounts that spread conspiracy theories.

These are certainly steps in the right direction, but research suggests that measures like fact-checking in politically polarized times face an uphill battle when it comes to actually changing minds. With our colleagues Diego Reinero, Elizabeth Harris, and Annie Duke, we recently ran experiments that pitted the power of fact-checks against social identity. Though they are usually less strong than true cult identities, we focused on people's connections to political parties. In the United States, more than 60 percent of people identify with one of the two major parties.

We had partisans on both sides read a series of statements that appeared to have come from Twitter. Each statement seemed to come from an in-group or an out-group member, and we asked participants how much they believed it was true. The statements looked like messages from political leaders, and we tried to capture some of the give-and-take that occurs during online political discussions.

For instance, participants might see a tweet that appeared to come from Donald Trump's Twitter account saying: "We were told that if global warming was real, the ice caps would be melting. However, they are now up at record levels." Then they saw this statement "fact-checked" by an in-group or out-group member. In this case, people in our study might have seen a response purportedly from Hillary Clinton noting: "According to the National Snow and Ice Data Center, the polar ice is at a record low in the Arctic (around the North Pole) right now and near record low in the Antarctic (around the South Pole). In no way are the caps at record highs." In other trials, participants saw prominent Democrats fact-checked by prominent Republicans, which allowed us to look at bias among supporters of both parties. Our question was, would fact-checks work, or would partisan identities dominate beliefs?

It turns out that fact-checks did work, but barely.

When people saw a post fact-checked, they tended to update their beliefs by very small amounts. For instance, if they believed Donald Trump's comment about global warming, they would report believing it about 1 percent less after reading Hillary Clinton's fact-check.

The dominant driver of beliefs, in our research, was whether the original tweet or the fact-check about it appeared to come from an in-group or an out-group member. People believed in-group members whether they were the ones who had shared the initial information or the fact-checking response. In this study, shared partisan reality was ten times more powerful than the fact-checks! And this was true for both Republicans and Democrats.

Our findings mesh with previous studies. It turns out that fact-checks work well for many topics, but not in the domain of politics. Once people have an identity at stake, the power of factual information is diluted—especially if it comes from the other side.

This is not terribly promising if we are hoping to reduce the influence and spread of erroneous information. Thankfully, other recent work suggests that there are techniques that can orient people more toward fact than fiction. Once again, a key factor turns out to be the goals with which people approach information. When people encounter something online, are they motivated to consider its accuracy or are they animated by another sort of goal—owning the libs, amusing their friends, or going viral?

To examine how different goals affect the processing of information online, researchers presented participants with a series of both true and false headlines about COVID-19 embedded in what looked like Facebook posts.[29] Half the participants were asked whether they would consider sharing each headline online; the other half were asked whether, to the best of their knowledge, the claim in each headline was accurate.

People who had been asked to consider accuracy discriminated between the true and false headlines significantly more effectively than those asked whether they would share the information. Focused on accuracy, people were better able to differentiate truth from lies. Research led by Steve Rathje and Sander van Linden similarly found that financial incentives can help reduce the spread of misinformation. Simply offering participants a dollar for forming accurate beliefs was sufficient to reduce their partisan biases.

When people want to be accurate, they are generally quite good at it. This places some power in our own hands. The challenge is how to create norms for accuracy in increasingly polarized environments where people often prefer to associate solely with like-minded others and take every opportunity to disagree with and disparage their perceived rivals.

And this raises the further challenge of how people who disagree due to their political commitments can work together. We offer a deeper understanding of this issue—as well as some potential solutions—in the next chapter.

CHAPTER 4

ESCAPING ECHO CHAMBERS

Imagine that you have been elected to your local city council and you want to figure out whether a potential new gun-control law banning concealed handguns would help reduce the city's crime rate. To determine if this type of legislation has a track record of success, you look at data from across the country, comparing cities that passed these laws in the preceding few years to cities that have not. You find that, among cities that did *not* ban concealed handguns, 225 experienced an increase in crime, while 75 saw their crime rates decrease. However, among cities that *did* ban concealed handguns, 105 experienced an increase in crime, while crime went down in 20.

Take a moment to crunch the numbers. Is this type of gun-control legislation effective?

Now imagine a different scenario. This time, you are working at a medical office and need to evaluate the efficacy of a new skin cream being sold as a cure for a nasty kind of rash. Once again, you do a comparison. Of patients who were *not* prescribed the new skin cream, 270 experienced a worsening of the rash, while 90 got better. Among patients who *did* use the new skin cream, 126 experienced a worsening of the rash and 24 got better.

Was this skin cream effective?

Now compare this answer to the previous question. Did you come to the same conclusion as you did for gun control?

The correct answers, based on these data (which are entirely hypothetical, by the way), is that neither the skin cream nor this gun-control legislation was effective. These questions are designed so that their answers are not obvious at a glance. But if you do the math, rashes improved among 25 percent of the patients who did *not* use the cream ($90 / [90 + 270] = .25$), but among only 16 percent of patients who did ($24 / [24 + 126] = .16$). Likewise, if you enter the numbers for gun control into the same equations, it reveals that crime rates decreased for 25 percent of cities without the gun-control legislation, but only 16 percent of cities that had enacted it. Expressed in reverse, the skin cream and the law were associated with worsening outcomes 84 percent of the time, while not using the cream and not enacting the law were associated with worsening outcomes only 75 percent of the time. Not a good skin cream and not a good law!

Although these two questions are mathematically identical, a funny thing happens when people complete them in research studies. A 2013 experiment by Yale law professor Dan Kahan and his colleagues found that American participants with reasonably good math skills tended to answer the question about the skin cream correctly. But when the question was about gun control, they often got it wrong.[1]

What's the difference? While skin care is a low-stakes issue for most people, gun control is not. In the United States particularly, any public policy involving guns tends to be a hotly contested political issue. When people answered the question about gun control, their math skills did not matter as much as their political identities. The mathematically correct answer about gun control should appeal to some partisans but dismay others. As a result, people whose political identities and beliefs aligned with the correct interpretation of these data were more likely to get the problem right.

Do you believe that gun control is effective and important? If so, you are less likely to have answered the question we gave you about gun control correctly. But if you do not believe in gun control, this question was likely easier for you. In fact, it probably felt like you knew the answer all along.

As we structured the question above, the right answer is that this particular gun-control law did not work—and in this case, Democrats in Kahan's study were less correct in their answers than Republicans. But as we said, the numbers in these questions are completely hypothetical and for other participants in the study, the correct answers were reversed. In that case, when the mathematically right answer was that gun control worked, Republicans were less likely to get it correct than Democrats.

Even among the most mathematically skilled participants in the study, partisans were 45 percent more likely to answer the gun-control question incorrectly when the right answer challenged their political beliefs. In short, their political identity seemed to make them dumber.

RISING PARTISANSHIP

Why does someone's political identity affect his or her ability to solve a math problem? The answer lies in a phenomenon that has become increasingly visible in public life: political partisanship. People identify with political leaders, parties, and belief systems, and these identities shape everything from how they apply their analytical skills in assessing public policies to voting behavior to dating.

In the political domain, the basic ingredients of social identity that we have discussed in this book can be amplified by sorting into highly competitive and oppositional political parties, by messages from partisan news sources, and by manipulation from political leaders and elites. The flow of information on social media also seems to play an increasingly important role.

At present, the United States, Canada, Britain, Brazil, Hungary, and many other countries around the world are experiencing intense political polarization.[2] In the U.S., this takes the form of conflict between Democrats on the left and Republicans on the right; in Britain, it recently manifested as conflict over the decision to leave or stay in the European Union (known as "Brexit"); in Brazil, it is reflected in support or opposition toward President Jair Bolsonaro, a divisive conservative leader. In Canada, liberals and conservatives have also become increasingly polarized, as they have in New Zealand, Switzerland, and other countries.

These trends have caused people to place greater emphasis on political identities than they used to, with effects on many aspects of their lives, from romance to how they project themselves on social media.[3] For instance, U.S. Twitter users are adding political words to their bios at a higher rate than words associated with any other social identity.[4] People are now more likely to describe themselves by their political affiliation than their religious affiliation. If we live in an age of identity, politics is increasingly the identity that matters for many people.

People spend less time together at Thanksgiving dinner if they disagree with their family members' politics.[5] Partisanship has even infiltrated romance.[6] Dating between members of different political parties is now more of a taboo among Americans than interracial dating. We ran a study on this around the time of Donald Trump's inauguration and found that fewer than one-quarter of people were willing to date someone from across the political aisle.[7]

Political disagreements and debates have always existed, and they are critical to healthy societies and robust democracies. But it is the nature of polarization to shift the psychology of social identity from in-group love (the normal sorts of preferences we have for our own groups) to out-group hate. Indeed, some political partisans may be more motivated by strong dislike of the opposition than by any special fondness for their own side. We hear people say that they are not voting for a candidate they like but *against* one whom they fear or despise.

Consistent with this, in the United States, survey data suggest that out-party hate has become more powerful than in-party love as a predictor of voting behavior.[8] This brand of hyper-oppositional political conflict includes worrying tendencies to view the other side as fundamentally different or alien to oneself, to strongly distrust the opposition and their intentions, and to view them as morally corrupt.

In this chapter, we explore the origins and dynamics of political conflict, how elements of the contemporary social environment have made it worse, and what we can do about it. Partisanship can lead people to reject evidence that is inconsistent with the party line or that discredits their leaders. And when entire groups of people deny facts in the service of partisan agendas, it can cause behaviors and policies that divide and damage societies. Our data and analyses are, admittedly, centered on the United States, but similar under-lying group dynamics are playing out in many nations.

POLITICAL BRAINS

The real problem of humanity is the following: We have paleolithic emotions, medieval institutions, and godlike technology.
—E. O. Wilson, "Looking Back, Looking Forward: A Conversation with James D. Watson and Edward O. Wilson"

Political differences have interesting links to human biology. Many people share the same policy preferences and party identification as their parents. We might expect that this is largely due to how they were raised, their views having been shaped by countless conversations around the dinner table. Many people assume that our politics are the product of social conditioning.

But it turns out that many of us are biologically predisposed to like certain parties and leaders. Research finds that nearly half of people's political beliefs have a genetic component. For instance, identical twins (who share 100 percent of their genetic material) are far more likely to share similar politics than nonidentical twins or siblings (who share a mere 50 percent).[9] Thus, if you split up identical twins as infants and placed one in a family of progressive liberals and the other in a family of staunch conservatives, there is a decent chance they would both eventually gravitate toward the same political party.

A few years ago, Oscar-winning actor Colin Firth speculated that liberals and conservatives must have different brains. He teamed up with a group of neuroscientists at University College London and together they launched a pair of studies in which they performed neuroimaging scans on the brains of a large number of liberals and conservatives.[10]

What they found was quite amazing. It turns out that they could predict people's political leanings with 72 percent accuracy simply by examining certain brain structures.

They looked at distinctions in the volume of gray matter that people had in different areas of the brain. Conservatives tended to have larger amygdalae; liberal participants tended to possess larger anterior cingulate cortices. Both regions are involved in a number of psychological processes, including how people react to emotional factors, social status, and conflict.

Mr. Firth is almost certainly the only person to win an Academy Award (Best Actor for *The King's Speech*) and publish a neuroscientific journal article in the same year. The research revealed clear neurological differences between people on different sides of the political spectrum and inspired our own foray into political neuroscience, further examining the particular role of the amygdala.

In a project led by Hannah Nam, Jay conducted a similar pair of studies at New York University with the aim of linking brain differences to actual political behavior. The research identified a similar pattern: slightly larger amygdalae in people who reported preferring the status quo to social change (a preference that is typically linked to conservatism).[11]

More important, though, we followed up a year later with the people whose brain structures we had measured to see if the size of this region predicted real political behavior. It did![12] We found that people with smaller amygdalae were more likely to have engaged in progressive liberal protests and collective action. In other words, people with less gray-matter density in this social-emotional brain region were more likely to report attending Black Lives Matter rallies, the March Against Climate Change, and even Occupy Wall Street.

What does this mean? It is not, of course, the case that people's genes or brains are preset to admire or endorse any particular politician, party, or policy. The specific political issues we grapple over in the twenty-first century—climate change, rights for members of sexual minority groups, minimum-wage hikes, and so on—are different from many of the concerns people had in the 1800s, let alone in the ancestral environments where humans evolved. What is more likely is that a person's biology predisposes him or her to experience the world in certain ways, ways that make specific political positions, parties, and leaders more or less appealing.

Conservatives, for example, tend to be more uncomfortable with change than liberals, preferring, all else being equal, that things remain the same.[13] They also tend to be more comfortable than liberals are with social hierarchies, preferring clear delineations of status and power. Both of these preferences probably have something of a biological basis, emerging from the ways that a person's nervous system responds to events. Some things feel more right or comfortable. Some situations cause more anxiety or concern. And these reactions to events orient the person toward different places on the political spectrum within their society.

People who enjoy change or who find flatter hierarchies and equity more pleasing find themselves more attracted to liberal positions. People who find change aversive or who want it to be clear who is in charge are drawn to more conservative positions.

The amygdala is a brain region involved in all sorts of emotional processes. Among other things, it has been linked to social hierarchies and social status in humans as well as in other species. In one brain-imaging study with humans, for example, the amygdala was involved when people learned about a new social hierarchy.[14] It is speculative, but people with more gray matter in this region may pay more attention to social rankings and, partially as a result, be more attracted to social arrangements that maintain hierarchies and policies that protect them.[15] Ultimately, they may be less willing to engage in activities that disrupt existing social arrangements, like protests.

As provocative as they are, biological differences like this are only part of the story. There is a chicken-or-egg problem with this type of brain data—we do not know if people's brain differences led to different political beliefs or if different types of political beliefs changed their brains.

More generally, while biological factors might attract people to certain types of politics, once they develop political identities, they look for cues about how to be good group members and filter events through the lens of that identity. People often sort themselves into groups of like-minded partisans, joining politically agreeable organizations, moving to more homogenous communities, and selectively tuning into certain brands of the evening news. And more recently, people have brought their politics online, where, it appears, partisan impulses often run wild.

ONLINE POLITICS

In the early days of the internet and social media, there was great excitement about the connective possibilities of these new technologies. Anyone could log on and interact not only with family and old friends but with a myriad of people from different backgrounds and cultures. These were to be portals to a new interconnected world in which humans could build a new sort of shared reality.

This much came true: we do live in a new world, more interconnected than at any point in history. The number of social media users around the globe, for example, totals well over four billion people.

But while people are certainly more connected in one sense, these technologies may have done just as much to divide them. They enable people to interact across cultures and borders, but they have also made it easier for people to seek out information that affirms their identities and confirms their beliefs. Instead of fostering human understanding, some social media companies have developed and monetized platforms and reward systems that facilitate some of the worst impulses of our partisan identities.

Research by our collaborator Molly Crockett has found that the internet is now a greater source of outrage for people than the lives they live offline.[16] Most of us rarely encounter immoral acts in our day-to-day physical lives. But online, it is another matter. In fact, people reported encountering more than three times as many immoral acts online as they do in print media, TV, and radio combined![17]

How often have you seen a person steal a purse or verbally assault someone? It happens, but in most places it is quite rare. However, on the internet, events like these are available for everyone and anyone to witness. The internet exposes users to a vast array of wicked acts, from neglectful parents or pet owners to bullying, corrupt politicians, and even the horrors of genocide.

The internet is a bottomless pit of depravity if you want it to be. You can log in and find enough immorality to keep your rage at a steady boil. As a result, people in Crockett's analysis reported experiencing significantly more outrage from online encounters than from interactions in any other part of their lives. Sadly, people also reported being significantly more likely to encounter information about immoral acts than about moral ones.

Negative reactions to events encountered online can have important and productive functions. Feelings of anger or guilt in response to injustices, for example, can motivate collective action. Twitter was credited with facilitating the Arab Spring uprisings in 2011, when citizens from countries across the Middle East and North Africa fought for greater freedoms from authoritarian regimes. Likewise, when people see videos of police brutality on Facebook or Twitter, it can move them to protest, run for political office, or fight for social change. We will discuss these dynamics of protest and change in more depth in chapter 7.

In many ways, these technologies have made people better informed than they were in the past. They have also helped people find like-minded others with whom they can form supportive communities that they might otherwise lack. The tremendous value of connective technologies like videoconferencing became particularly apparent during the COVID-19 pandemic, which forced people everywhere to separate physically. Suddenly the two of us were teaching entirely online. Our scientific conferences shifted to virtual venues. And we coordinated much of the writing of this book via text message, exchanging thousands of thoughts as they occurred to us.

But there is a growing awareness that these technological innovations, and social media in particular, have a dark side.

INSIDE THE ECHO CHAMBER

"Join us in the streets! Stop Trump and his bigoted agenda!" read an announcement on the Black Matters U.S. Facebook page. The rally attracted roughly ten thousand protesters, who marched from Union Square, a few blocks from Jay's apartment in New York City, to the gilded entrance of Trump Tower near the southern edge of Central Park.

Around the same time, in the run-up to the 2016 presidential election, the Florida Goes Trump organization arranged rallies in more than twenty cities across the Sunshine State. News releases touting these events were ripped straight from Trump's stump speeches, encouraging "patriots" to help "Make America Great Again!"

Although these initiatives had the rhythm and cadence of grass-roots political events, they actually had far more sinister origins. In a legal indictment, special counsel Robert Mueller later revealed that both of these organizations were fronts for a massive Russian scheme to manipulate the election and disrupt the democratic process. In particular, the Russians sought to turn Americans against one another by appealing to their political identities.

Throughout the election season, Russian propagandists ran divisive ads on Facebook and posted content on Twitter targeting issues such as gun control, civil rights, and fears about "the other," including immigrants and Muslims. In one message, Hillary Clinton's head, complete with red horns, was photoshopped onto the body of a devil as she squared off to fight Jesus. The headline " 'Like' if You Want Jesus to Win!" was plastered at the top of the image, with the words *Army of Jesus* in small print at the bottom. Facebook estimates that up to one hundred fifty million people saw ads like this in the months leading up to the 2016 election.

It was obvious that these ads were memes designed to appeal to and inflame partisan conflict. The messages included potent symbols of American identity: the Stars and Stripes, cowboys, even a heroic cartoon of a chiseled Bernie Sanders wearing nothing more than a red Speedo.

This disinformation campaign was not simply a matter of spreading falsehoods that could be rooted out with fact-checking—these ads were designed to drive a wedge between Americans. Russian propaganda usually brings to mind Cold War–era images of Stalin and Lenin towering over brigades of soldiers or rows of missiles, but propagandized memes in the age of Facebook and Twitter are different, rich with the language and imagery of contemporary social identities. And these messages tend to get amplified by the most extreme partisans.

There has been a great deal of concern recently about how algorithms on social media platforms might be creating "filter bubbles," in which people are largely shown news, opinions, and memes that are consistent with their beliefs. Facebook and YouTube want to give users maximally pleasant experiences online, so news feeds and recommended videos may avoid exposing people to things they do not want to know. Worse, certain kinds of algorithms can lead people down rabbit holes into increasingly extreme information environments.

It is not clear how much of a problem this actually is. It is hard to pin down exactly what platforms' algorithms are doing, partly because the mechanics behind these algorithms are hidden from the public, partly because they change all the time, and partly because different platforms do different things. And it is certainly the case that social media companies, especially the large ones, have become more attentive to the potential problems of filter bubbles and radicalization. However, the sorts of psychological and identity-related dynamics we have discussed in earlier chapters point to a variety of ways that people can be led into belief-confirming information bubbles even without the input of social media algorithms.

People often selectively affiliate with those who are similar to themselves, maintaining connections to people they agree with and blocking or un-friending everyone else. Further, even if their media feeds contain a diversity of perspectives, they may selectively pay attention to and remember identity-consistent information—the "facts" that confirm their social realities. They are more attuned to in-group norms and likely to let the consensus among like-minded people shape their own opinions on issues. And they may seek to signal these identities to the world by sharing and resharing identity-consistent information.

In the social media age, conversations about political, social, and cultural issues have moved from discussions among family at the dinner table or friends at the local tavern to a much wider public sphere. This shift has allowed researchers like us to analyze some of the psychological elements driving political discourse on a massive scale. We have started to examine how identities get expressed on-line and how divisive language can foster intergroup conflict (and vice versa).

People are now bombarded with information. By one estimate, the average social media user scrolls through more than three hundred feet of content every day.[18] If you own a six-inch smart-phone, this means you swipe your screen about six hundred times a day on one social media platform or another—roughly the equivalent of scrolling down the length of the Statue of Liberty, inch by inch.

To examine how people filter this overwhelming amount of information, Jay and his former students Billy Brady and Ana Gant-man ran laboratory experiments using classic measures of attention to see what kinds of messages would jump out at people.[19] Partici-pants saw words and messages streaming across a computer screen similar to what they see while scrolling through their social media feeds. The words varied in content. Some were fairly neutral in tone (for example, *thing, motorcycle*), while others were much more emotional or moralistic (*weep, pure, holy, afraid*). Perhaps unsurprisingly, people's attention was captured more readily by emotional and moral words than by neutral ones. We reasoned that this may be how the attention economy works, by grabbing viewers' attention with visceral language, which might lead them to share those messages with their own social networks.

To test this, we analyzed a large sample of more than half a million real messages on Twitter with content related to contentious political topics, including gun control, same-sex marriage, and climate change. Sure enough, we found that the same sorts of words that had captured our participants' attention in the lab were also more likely to be shared by real users on Twitter.

We found that for each moral-emotional word included in a tweet, the chance that another person would retweet that message increased by roughly 15 percent. Interestingly, purely moral words (like *mercy* and *right*) or purely emotional words (like *afraid* and *love*) didn't have the same impact. It was words that combined moral connotations with emotional reactions—words like *hate, shame,* and *ruin*—that packed the biggest punch.

We also found that the more moral-emotional words people used in a message, the more likely it was to spread beyond their followers. If someone jammed four or five of these words in a tweet, it was likely to spread even further. People typically retweet messages to their social network because they endorse the content and trust the source. But moral-emotional words appear to add rocket fuel to this decision. Messages go viral when they capture attention.

A cheeky student at another university read our paper about this study and decided to compose a tweet consisting almost entirely of the fifteen most powerful moral-emotional words: *attack, bad, blame, care, destroy, fight, hate, kill, murder, peace, safe, shame, terrorism, war,* and *wrong*. As if to prove our point, his message was quickly shared more than eight hundred times and liked by another seventeen hundred individuals! Even in jest, certain words have power.

This pattern of moral contagion was observed in every topic we

THE POWER OF US

studied, from climate change to gun control. We found the same pattern for people on the left and the right (though the effect was slightly stronger on the right), on different social media platforms, and among political leaders and regular citizens. It also held for people with large or small social networks and for positive or negative messages. Whether people were talking about honor or hatred, moral-emotional language resonated far beyond their immediate social networks.

If you are hoping to go viral, you might be thinking about using these sorts of words in your next social media post. But we should warn you that, while they can inspire your in-group, they might well alienate people on the other side. Indeed, that may often be the point.

SOWING DIVISION

> I think social media has more power than the
> money they spent.
>
> —Donald Trump, *60 Minutes*

Many political leaders and their advisers understand the power of evocative language on social media. It's hard to find a better example of this than Donald Trump, who tweeted extensively throughout his campaign and one-term presidency (until ultimately being banned from Twitter after the January 6, 2021, insurrection due to "the risk of further incitement of violence"). In his first national interview after winning the 2016 election, Trump claimed that social media had helped make up for the fact that the Clinton campaign outspent his by roughly five hundred million dollars.[20] But what did he do to harness the power of social media?

To find out, we analyzed how he and other political leaders used Twitter.

In a project led by Billy Brady, we examined the Twitter accounts of every American political leader elected to federal office in 2016. In the year leading up their elections, these officials had posted a whopping 286,255 messages on the platform.[21] Although many of these politicians presumably had staffers to help manage their online messaging, we nevertheless found the same pattern as among everyday citizens: the use of moral-emotional language was one of the best predictors of whether their messages went viral.

From the least prominent congressional candidates to well-known senators, the average politician saw more than a 10 percent increase in retweets for every moral-emotional word used in a message. One of the most notable beneficiaries was, of course, Donald Trump. When we analyzed Trump's account, we found that every moral-emotional word he used increased the chance of his message being retweeted by 25 percent. In his case, we are talking about messages that were being retweeted tens of thousands of times and driving discussion—and sometimes policy—on national and international issues.

When we looked more closely at Trump's most viral messages, we saw they tended to include the language of collective victimization. Words like *blamed, brutal, hurt, abandon, victims, steal, abuse,* and *guilty* were among the most powerful terms he used in the year leading up to the election. Playing the victim was an effective tool for spreading his gospel.

We suspect this language was designed to mobilize his supporters while sowing divisions within the rest of the country. Making the people in your group feel that they have been attacked creates the perception that you are all under threat, and when this is done via social media, it serves as a cheap and powerful strategy to generate a shared sense of identity.

Despite their potential to go viral, however, retweets inspired by partisan language rarely crossed ideological lines. We were able to estimate the political identities and ideologies of a sample of Twitter users by examining whom they followed and who followed them.

For instance, if you followed Hillary Clinton and Barack Obama, you were more likely to be a liberal/Democrat; if you followed Donald Trump and Mitt Romney, you were more likely to be a conservative/ Republican. If you followed all of them, you were likely to be a moderate, a member of the press corps, or just confused!

In the analysis of tweets by ordinary citizens that we described above, we found that when they used and responded to moral-emotional language, they ended up in disconnected echo chambers. Liberals tended to retweet messages from other liberals and conservatives from other conservatives. While messages with moral emotions spread like wildfire within these groups, they rarely seemed to appeal to people across the political divide.

Of course, some tweets do more than just deploy highly charged words; they actively derogate the other side. We recently analyzed this type of hyper-oppositional language on Twitter and Facebook in a project led by colleagues Steve Rathje and Sander van Linden. This time, we were able to examine more than 2.7 million messages across these platforms.

Every time a negative message described an out-group member, it was associated with a massive increase in sharing. And when these messages came from a congressperson's account, the out-group-directed message increased sharing by up to 180 percent, dwarfing the impact of moral-emotional language on its own. On Facebook, posts about the out-group also elicited the most angry reactions, fueling the expressions of moral outrage that now dominate so much of political discourse online.

It is tempting to discount online conversations as not being "real life." But any divide between life online and life in the real world has become so blurred as to be nearly meaningless. Online activity drives real-world behavior, and activity on social media is increasingly leaking into real life. For instance, one analysis by Marlon Mooijman and his colleagues found that the hourly frequency of moralized tweets during anti-police protests predicted later numbers of arrests during protests, suggesting that online moralization was associated with and might have been a contributor to conflict on the streets.[22]

Divisive language can be highly rewarded on social media, in part due to platform design. On Facebook or Twitter, you can Like comments that you appreciate with the click of a button, while it takes more effort to register your disdain. Thus, when people post provocative content, they readily see affirmation from like-minded partisans, while reservations that their friends and families might hold are harder to register. The system reinforces people's more extreme expressions of opinion and obscures the disdain or eye-rolls that would normally accompany those same statements if they were made at work or over dinner. This incentive structure may increase engagement and profits for social media giants, but it can lead citizens further down the path of intergroup separation and conflict.

In fact, when we ran a series of lab experiments using disagreeable Twitter messages, we found that people did not want to have a conversation about politics with someone from the other side who used moral-emotional language. They found the comments off-putting and concluded that the message was crafted from someone with a closed mind. This was especially true of people who had the strongest sense of identification with their political party.[23]

But when people disagreed using less highly charged language, it created an opportunity for dialogue across partisan divides. People are sometimes willing to engage with others on difficult issues, but only when their differences are framed in ways that do not automatically imply that one or the other side is immoral.

Of course, inflammatory language and increasingly separated social networks are not the only problem—or even the most important problem—for politics online. Mis- and disinformation are challenging democratic societies everywhere. And when people possess strong political identities, they may be more vulnerable to false facts, increasing their willingness to believe—and share—factually flawed information that casts opponents in a negative light.

FAKE NEWS!

Remember the Russian propagandists posting polarizing ads on social media? It turns out that this was only the tip of the iceberg in terms of mis- and disinformation during the run-up to the 2016 presidential election. From Macedonia to Michigan, people were generating and sharing fake news stories to manipulate and confuse U.S. voters.

One study estimated that up to 44 percent of adult Americans visited an untrustworthy website in the final weeks before the election, and millions more saw this type of content in their social media feeds.[24] Nearly a quarter of Americans reported sharing a made-up news story, and recent research suggests that partisans often think that sharing fake news is morally permissible. Some people knew the stories were dubious, but others might have been fooled because they wanted to believe. One single fake news story, published by a site called WTOE 5 News, reported that Pope Francis had broken with tradition and endorsed Donald Trump for president. This phony story received nearly a million endorsements on Facebook, roughly three times as many as the top story from the *New York Times*!

Similar waves of fake news washed over other countries, including Britain during the 2016 Brexit vote and Brazil during its national election in 2018. This is an international epidemic. Social media companies and scientists alike have been scrambling ever since to try to understand how and why people spread, and often believe, false facts.

Just as in cults, ordinary citizens look to fellow group members—especially group leaders—to help determine their beliefs. Finding news that affirms their most cherished identities can help people feel a sense of superiority, provide a story to bond over, or reinforce a sense that they are on the right side of history. By fulfilling core social needs and aligning with their prior beliefs, certain news stories are appealing regardless of their veracity. This may explain why the most popular fake news stories highlight the virtues of one group over another. When the pope bestows his fictitious endorsement on Donald Trump, for example, it provides a feeling of reinforcement for conservative Catholics and other Christians who want to feel principled about their political preferences.

The problem is that these social motives and beliefs can outweigh the desire for accuracy, causing people to be overly credulous when it comes to identity-affirming information. We have conducted several studies in which we found that people tend to believe positive stories about their in-groups and negative stories about out-groups, no matter how dubious the information may be.

In a series of experiments led by Andrea Pereira and Elizabeth Harris, we presented real and fake news stories to 1,420 Americans to see how their political identities shaped their reactions.[25] Some of these articles were negative fake news stories about Democrats. One headline, for example, claimed that "Hillary Wore Secret Ear-Piece During Debate" and another that "Florida Democrats Just Voted to Impose Sharia Law on Women." Other articles contained negative fake news stories about Republicans, like one claiming "President Trump Enacts One-Child Law for Minorities."

We sampled these stories from actual fake or satirical news websites. We found that Republicans were more willing to believe nasty fake news stories about Democrats than about Republicans. Similarly, Democrats were more willing to believe fake news stories about Republicans than about Democrats. To make matters worse, participants' belief in a fake news story was a powerful predictor of their willingness to share it on social media. The findings were strikingly similar across parties: Democrats and Republicans alike had a blind spot for fake news about the other side.

Skeptics will point out that because we harvested these stories from actual websites, there might have been differences between the stories about Democrats and Republicans. Perhaps one type of fake story was more believable than the other. We had the same concern, so we reran the study but created our own damaging fake news articles that were identical in every detail except whether the target was a Republican or a Democrat.

In this study, people read about a Democrat or Republican who was corrupt in precisely the same way. This study replicated our original results almost exactly, showing again that Republicans and Democrats were guided by their identities to believe bad news about the out-group.

This doesn't mean there were no differences between the left and the right. One difference was in terms of who was more willing to share fake news with their social networks. While Democrats and Republicans were equally likely to believe fake news about the other side, Republicans were more willing to share it with their friends and family. This might explain why stories like the one about the pope endorsing Trump went viral during the 2016 election cycle.

We do not know exactly why Republicans were more willing to share these stories, but it seems plausible that their party might have had more lenient norms about sharing fake news. Trump himself was a super-spreader of misinformation, and this might have signaled to his supporters that they could place more trust in low-quality news sources or that it was fine to share sketchy information.

We also found a difference in how much partisans on the left and the right believed fake news that had nothing to do with politics. When we gave people false information unrelated to politics— like articles about the British royal Camilla, Duchess of Cornwall, going to rehab or celebrity Leonardo DiCaprio flying an eyebrow artist 7,500 miles to sculpt his handsome brows—Republicans were more willing to believe this as well. It seemed that Democrats were generally more skeptical about fake news unless it was negative news about Republicans, whereas Republicans were generally more likely to believe fake news about a variety of topics.

A great deal of mis- and disinformation spreads on social media platforms and it's easy to place blame for the resulting political polarization on social media. But these technologies are far from the only way that people end up in ideological cocoons. People can subscribe to a newspaper that bends over backward to affirm its readers' identities, tune into a news station that feeds them an unhealthy dose of groupthink, or watch their favorite television host foam at the mouth every night before bed. Social media gets lots of the blame but it is only a modest part of the story, which may explain why older people, who have consumed a steady diet of increasingly partisan news for years, are far more polarized than the millennials who grew up on social media. Indeed, some experts believe that the polarization of the mainstream media has been more divisive than the rise of social media.

A phrase famously attributed to Daniel Patrick Moynihan states, "Everyone is entitled to his own opinion, but not his own facts." Our research suggests that this is wishful thinking when it comes to political partisans. In the contemporary political landscape, comedian Stephen Colbert was closer to the truth when he said in an interview with the *AV Club*, "It used to be everyone was entitled to their own opinion, but not their own facts. But that's not the case anymore. Facts matter not at all. Perception is everything." This is not a good thing because facts do, indeed, still matter. Reality can come back to bite us.

A PARTISAN PANDEMIC

During the early stages of the COVID-19 pandemic, there was no vaccine or medical treatment. Public health experts around the world declared that one of the most important ways to slow the virus was for people to maintain physical distance from one another. For many, this meant staying home as much as possible and dramatically curtailing their patterns of movement. But as officials implored people to stay home and avoid crowds, media images of parties, pub crawls, and packed beaches suggested that these messages were not being heeded by everyone.

There are numerous reasons people might have ignored the advice of public health experts, ranging from the overconfidence of youth to conspiracy theories. But in the United States especially, polls suggested that a partisan divide was partly to blame. An NBC News/*Wall Street Journal* poll conducted in early March 2020 found that while 68 percent of Democrats were worried that someone in their family could catch the virus, just 40 percent of Republicans were worried. Another poll reported that Democrats were 18 percent more likely to avoid large crowds than Republicans were.[26]

Why was there such a large partisan gap in concerns about the virus? One possibility is that many conservatives live in more rural, less dense neighborhoods, and many liberals live in cities, which are large and crowded and provide optimal conditions for the virus to spread. Indeed, Jay spent the first few months of the pandemic hunkered down in Manhattan when it was a global hot spot.

But another potential explanation was the dynamics of political identity. Leaders and elites associated with the two parties were sending different messages, which might have shaped their followers' perceptions of the risks. Prominent voices on the right were openly skeptical about the pandemic. Fox News host Sean Hannity said on his WOR talk-radio program that it may be true that the coronavirus issue was a "fraud" spread by the "deep state," and his colleague at Fox Trish Regan accused Democrats of using the coronavirus crisis "to destroy and demonize this President."[27]

Indeed, the most influential member of the Republican Party, President Trump, was one of the fiercest pandemic skeptics. He initially called concerns about the pandemic a "Democratic hoax" and consistently downplayed the risks of the virus, as well as the importance and effectiveness of measures like distancing.[28]

To see if partisan attitudes toward the virus were mirrored in real behavior, not just in opinion polls, we examined the physical movement of people in Republican versus Democratic counties and states across the United States.[29] We joined forces with Anton Gollwitzer and his colleagues at Yale University and analyzed geo-tracking data from over seventeen million smartphone users to see if people from politically divergent locations engaged in different physical-distancing behaviors. To protect anonymity, we did not use individual smartphone data but looked at levels of movement in entire counties.

The results were startlingly clear. From March 9 to May 8, during the first spike of the pandemic, blue-county citizens stayed home and red-county citizens kept moving. Overall, U.S. counties that voted for Donald Trump over Hillary Clinton in 2016 exhibited 16 percent more movement as well as more visits to nonessential services like restaurants. To be fair, everyone began to distance more and engage in less nonessential movement as the pandemic spread, but as this happened, the partisan gap only increased!

We tested a number of potential explanations. It turns out the partisan gap in movement could not be explained by population density, local rates of COVID-19 infections, economic factors like household incomes and employment rates, or the average age and religious affiliation of the population. Instead, the amount of conservative-media consumption in each county accounted for less physical distancing among the people living there. In other words, the more conservative news consumed, the more people kept moving.

During a deadly pandemic, these partisan differences were anything but trivial. When we analyzed infection and mortality rates, we found that less physical distancing in Republican counties was associated with an increased growth rate in COVID-19 infections and fatalities two weeks later.

This devastating discrepancy did not have to be the case. If Americans had peeked across the border to Canada, they would have observed a different dynamic. Researchers there found no evidence of political leaders from any political party downplaying the pandemic. As a consequence, Canadians exhibited no political differences in terms of physical distancing. This does not mean that Canadians are fundamentally different from their American friends to the south. Rather, leaders and elites in the two countries provided very different cues about what to believe, with real impacts on the behavior and the lives of citizens.

By shaping how people see themselves and what they believe about the world, effective leaders have the ability to bring people together to tackle national and global challenges. One of the best examples of this form of leadership during the pandemic was from New Zealand's prime minister, Jacinda Ardern. She not only closely followed the advice of scientists in facing the pandemic but helped inspire her citizens to follow the guidelines. She did this by creating a shared sense of identity, calling them her "team of 5 million" and clearly following the guidelines herself.[30] (We will talk much more about the relationship between identity and leadership in chapter 9.)

The way that people moved around during the COVID-19 pandemic was one manifestation of a relationship between politics and space. More generally, political differences can cause people to physically separate from one another, and, as it turns out, physical separations might further drive political differences.

CROSSING THE AISLE

It was a classic rookie mistake. On January 3, 2019, his first day in office, Andy Kim walked into the House Chamber in Washington, DC, and sat himself down. Normally there would be nothing controversial about taking a seat, but the newly elected congressperson for New Jersey's Third District had unknowingly seated himself in the Republican section of the House. And he was a Democrat.

"I was just looking around for a seat," Kim later reported.[31]

Except that here, in one of the most polarized spaces in the world, a seat is not just a seat. One side of the House Chamber is designated seating for Republicans and the other side is designated for Democrats. The seats are powerful symbols of partisan allegiances. They demark where people belong and, generally speaking, are a pretty good indicator of what people believe. As Truman-era civil servant Rufus Miles put it: "Where you stand depends on where you sit."

Few places are as sharply or spatially divided as the U.S. Congress, although the consequences for Andy Kim weren't as bad as they might have been for a fan who sits in the wrong section of some European soccer stadiums. Rifts in space signal and reinforce differences in social identity.

However, Congress is a workplace where people with different political views and party affiliations must interact in order to achieve important objectives. Politicians often need to cross the aisle to broker compromise and pass new laws. Yet people are physically sorted on the basis of their political views. If people need to interact with one another to get things done, does this spatial sorting pose a hindrance to American governance?

Researchers recently applied motion-detection technology to 6,526 videos of Congress in action to examine how Republicans and Democrats moved around the chamber.[32] How many times did they literally cross the aisle? As you might expect, Democrats and Republicans were less likely to cross the aisle that divides the middle

117

of Congress than they were to move about in proximity to members of their own party.

More worrisome, however, this trend increased over time. Between January 1997 and December 2012, as the two parties became more polarized in their political preferences, the videos revealed less commingling between members of the two parties after floor votes. Congresspeople spent less time physically interacting with members of the other party.

It is natural to assume that partisan votes might have reduced interaction. But the timing of the pattern suggested it was the other way around—a lack of physical interaction was associated with more polarized voting behavior in the future. Reducing informal interactions might have made it harder to form the friendships and bonds across the aisle that make bipartisan legislation possible, leading to less cooperative voting patterns over time. A lack of interaction might also have made it harder to understand the perspectives of the other side.

Given all of these challenges, then, what might be done?

SEEKING ANTIDOTES

Researchers, policy makers, politicians, and social media executives everywhere are scrambling not only to understand how technological advances are affecting civic life but also to find ways to reduce some of the harms they have caused. There has been an explosion of research on these issues, and new studies come out every day.

It is tempting to think that the solution to echo chambers and filter bubbles is simply to provide people with a more diverse diet of information, exposing them to views and perspectives from the other side. This type of approach assumes that the underlying problem is a knowledge deficit and that if people were only better informed or educated about issues, all would be well. Unfortunately, however, it seems that gaining more knowledge about politics and simply being exposed to a broader array of information is not necessarily going to help.

Can receiving information from outside your partisan echo chamber help reduce political divisions? Sociologist Christopher Bail and his colleagues tested this possibility in a large field experiment. They offered groups of Democrats and Republicans eleven dollars each to follow a Twitter bot that retweeted twenty-four political messages every day for a month.[33] Critically, the bot was always of a different ideological persuasion than the participant, and it randomly sent them tweets from accounts belonging to elected officials, opinion leaders, media organizations, and nonprofits on the other side.

Unfortunately, receiving tweets from sources across the political aisle did absolutely nothing to soften political attitudes. In fact, it backfired. Democrats' attitudes became more liberal after following a conservative account, and Republicans' attitudes became more conservative after following a liberal account. Simply getting different information is not enough, in part because people are often motivated to dismiss and argue against messages they know are coming from the other side.

An antidote to this could be to remove partisan identity from the equation. One study found, for example, that people can effectively learn about polarized issues like climate change from interacting with partisans on the opposing side as long as social identities remain in the background.[34] People were presented with a graph from NASA illustrating the average monthly level of Arctic sea ice over the past thirty-four years. The long-term trend was clearly one of steadily reducing ice, but the most recent year shown on the graph exhibited a modest increase in ice levels. They were then asked to forecast the amount of Arctic sea ice that would be left by 2025.

After reviewing the chart, conservatives were significantly less likely than liberals to interpret the NASA graph in a manner consistent with the long-term trend. But all participants then had a chance to update and potentially improve their estimates by viewing other people's responses. Exposure to a bipartisan set of responses, rather than responses only from one's own side, improved everyone's estimate. However, the ability to learn from others with different perspectives was significantly smaller if people's party identity or logo was attached to their responses. But if party logos were removed and political identities were hidden, people were more influenced by others and improved their own estimates by nearly 20 percent.

Society might be better served if political symbols were removed from news reports and interviews; this might focus audiences on details of policy proposals rather than partisan loyalties. In normal conversation, people often lead with their identities. This can promote transparency and provide standing on certain issues, but it may also close minds and foster disagreement. We might want to think twice before invoking our political identities if we're aiming to talk across a divide.

Recent research further suggests that while simply receiving information from political out-groups is not necessarily an effective strategy for tackling polarization, actual interactions between people with different points of view can help. In a recent study, Erin Rossiter randomly assigned a set of Republicans and Democrats to engage in short online chats about political or nonpolitical topics.[35] Regardless of what they talked about, participants who had engaged in digital communication with a political out-group member later felt more positively toward the out-group than people who had not had these conversations.

Leaving the online sphere entirely, at least for a time, might also help. In one study done in the fall of 2018, economists encouraged people (sometimes by offering them money) to disconnect from their Facebook accounts for a month.[36] Over the course of the month, these people spent less time online and experienced an increase in psychological well-being. They also became less knowledgeable about the news and less politically polarized. Remarkably, the reduction in polarized attitudes observed in a single month was equivalent to about half the total amount that polarization has increased in the United States since the mid-1990s!

Finally, it may be helpful to draw people's attention more precisely to just how polarized our societies actually are. As we mentioned above, polarization has increased in many places. This is especially true among elites like politicians. Among ordinary citizens, however, it is a bit more complicated. Populations at large are experiencing high levels of what has been called "affective," or emotional, polarization, with people holding strong feelings of distrust and dislike for political out-groups. When researchers look at people's opinions on actual issues and policies, however, they tend to find less evidence of polarization.

Certainly there are differences of opinion, but large majorities of people on the left and the right are often fairly close in their attitudes toward even controversial issues. In the United States, for example, people on the left and right are not very far apart in their opinions about health care, certain kinds of gun control, and immigration. Overestimating how much we differ may be an impediment to even trying to reach a compromise. And yet, most of the information people get about politics reinforces the idea of unbridgeable divides. Even the way electoral maps are presented, for example, gives the impression of nations sharply split.

On election night, we are used to seeing maps of the country showing how people in different places voted. In the United States, these maps indicate red Republican states and blue Democratic states. They give the impression of unanimity within each state. But in reality, of course, every state contains a mix of people, and in some cases, the number of people voting for each party's candidate may actually be very close. A more accurate depiction of voters' preferences would show different shades of colors—more red for states with more Republican votes, more blue for states with more Democrats, and many shades of purple in between.

A study by Sara Konrath and colleagues showed people precisely these kinds of more proportionally accurate and quite purple maps.[37] Compared with people who saw the standard red and blue, these participants subsequently stereotyped their political out-groups less and saw the United States as less divided. Similarly, shattering the stereotypes people have about members of the other party can pave the way for more positive interactions.

As we said, a great deal of research attention is being dedicated to tackling political divisions and their sources online. As consumers of information and as group members themselves, people can use strategies to try to come to less biased and more accurate understandings of issues. Research has found that when people take the time to reason systematically rather than going with their gut intuitions, they are less likely to get suckered into believing fake political news. Deliberate and critical thinking can help people win the tug-of-war between partisan goals and accuracy goals.

Give yourself time to stop and carefully consider the reputability of the source of a news article before you share it with others. Be wary if a story that is damaging to the other side seems too good to be true; those feelings of glee might be a tip-off that you want to believe it, not that you actually do. Consider tuning out distractions from your phone or e-mail the next time you engage with a story about politics. Simply being distracted can reduce your ability to reason carefully about the news. In a project with our collaborators at Cambridge University, we found that increasing accuracy motives can have the same effect; offering people a small incentive for accurate judgments reduces polarization in responses to inaccurate information.

Warning others that they might have been presented with misinformation can also help. In your own groups, try to make fact-checking and questioning assumptions a valued part of the norms and identity. Build an identity grounded in accuracy and constructive feedback.

When you are talking to people across the aisle, try to understand that their identity motives and beliefs might be getting in the way of their seeing your perspective. Remove symbols of identity. If that is not possible, you might be able to frame the issue in language that resonates with their identity and values or at least that acknowledges how meaningful their identity is to them.

We have a long way to go to solve the problems of partisanship while promoting healthy debate over serious issues. But understanding the identity dynamics that underlie these divisions provides a foundation for healthier political spheres where the focus can stay more squarely on the serious matters that affect the lives and well-being of citizens.

CHAPTER 5

THE VALUE OF IDENTITY

"What is truly Scandinavian? Absolutely nothing" ran a provocative ad promoting Scandinavian Airlines in 2020.[1]

Many Scandinavians were not amused. Although Scandinavian Airlines has been described as "an icon of Norwegian-Swedish-Danish cooperation," their ad somehow managed to unite citizens of these three countries in sharp criticism of the company.

The ad described how things that are globally considered staples of Nordic identity, like Danish pastries and Swedish meatballs, were all invented elsewhere. It showed citizens from these countries looking depressed and forlorn as they learn that various sources of national and regional pride were, well, ripped off from entrepreneurs, inventors, and civil rights leaders in other nations.

"We take everything we like from our trips abroad, adjust it a little bit, and *voilà!* It's a unique Scandinavian thing." The ad concluded with the suggestion that travel enriches these countries' citizens and their cultural heritage, and hence true Scandinavians should purchase airline tickets forthwith and go out to explore the world.

As an attempt at identity-based inspiration, the ad was a woeful failure. It managed to foster a degree of public outrage toward an airline advertisement that is probably unprecedented. Several conservative politicians swore never to fly with them again. And the reaction was magnified by thousands of citizens on social media. When we watched the ad on YouTube, it had over 131,000 thumbs-down symbols, more than ten times the number of people who gave it a thumbs-up.

Company officials eventually pulled the ad and said they were proud of their Scandinavian heritage. They regretted that their message had been misunderstood.[2] But how could a company blow a message about identity this badly? And what does it take to get it right? Across the Atlantic Ocean, a beer company offered the answers to some of these questions.

Wearing a plaid shirt and faded blue jeans, Jeff Douglas strode onto the stage and approached the microphone. He quietly began speaking to the people in the theater, hesitantly at first. "Hey, I'm not a lumberjack or a fur trader and I don't live in an igloo or eat blubber or own a dogsled and I don't know Jimmy, Sally, or Susie from Canada, although I'm certain they're really, really nice."

He raised his voice slowly as he continued. "I have a prime minister, not a president. I speak English and French, not American, and I pronounce it 'about,' not 'a boot.'" Footage showing beavers, a chesterfield, the letter Z (pronounced "zed"), and a toque (a knitted winter hat) played on a large screen behind him.

Now reaching a roar, he declared, "Canada is the second-largest landmass, the first nation in hockey, and the best part of North America," as highlights from a classic hockey game and an image of a massive Canadian flag rolled on the screen. Then, in climax: "My name is Joe and I am Canadian."

This speech, known affectionately as "the rant," lasted just a minute.[3] But it became the centerpiece of one of the most successful beer-advertising campaigns in Canadian history. It was part of the "I am Canadian" campaign launched in the year 2000 by Molson Breweries, the oldest brewing company in Canada. The savvy marketing team knew that Molson's most important ingredient wasn't the hops in their beer but the company's identity.

The rant was a bald attempt to sell beer using nationalism, and the beer they were advertising was already named Canadian. Yet it helped articulate something that many felt was missing from the national conversation. It is fair to say that Canadians are often shy about expressing their national identity in such a bold way. But characterizing what it means to be Canadian, especially in contrast to its bigger, more powerful neighbor to the south, allowed Canadians to define who they were.

Every Canadian who wore a toque, owned a chesterfield, or pronounced the letter *Z* as "zed" felt a sense not only of *belonging* but also of *distinctiveness.* It was the very opposite of the Scandinavian Airlines ad, which managed to neglect the sense of belonging people desire and undercut any feelings of distinctiveness. That deflating ad was almost perfectly crafted to threaten people's cultural identity rather than affirm it.

By combining these two psychological ingredients, belonging plus distinctiveness, the "I am Canadian" campaign resonated with Canadians. It launched a banner year for Molson Breweries, seeing the company gain 1.6 points on the stock market. This unadorned attempt to market a social identity was clearly enough to sell cases— many, many cases—of Molson Canadian beer.

But the rant did more than move beer; it moved people in a way that a beer commercial rarely does. The rant received the Gold Quill Award from the advertising industry in 2001 and was imitated and parodied across Canada. It was even included in the *Penguin Treasury of Popular Canadian Poems and Songs* because, as John Colombo, editor of the collection, put it, the words "express a human need to affirm an identity in the face of ignorance and indifference."

The rant signifies the power of identity to shape the value we place on everything from products to people. People often think that their tastes are a unique part of their individuality. Indeed, they often want to be distinctive with their own idiosyncratic set of preferences. Ask your friend why she drinks a certain brand of beer and we doubt she will say it is because she identifies with the brewery.

But aspects of one's identity have an influence on all sorts of daily decisions, often outside one's conscious awareness. Your preferences are fundamentally shaped by your social identity, and the reason is quite simple: your social identity is you. In this chapter, we explain how different motives shape identity, focusing particularly on core human needs for belonging, distinctiveness, and status. These motives make certain identities more attractive and important and, in turn, shape how people value individuals and things in the world around them. From the foods people eat to whom they choose to date to the products they buy to the schools they attend, identity is at the heart of many of their most important decisions.

IDENTITY ECONOMICS

We are hardly alone in the opinion that identities matter deeply for decisions. Nobel laureate George Akerlof and Rachel Kranton wrote an entire book, called *Identity Economics,* in which they claim that the "choice of identity…may be the most important economic decision a person ever makes."[4] Once we understand how identity influences value, we can see why some decisions that might seem irrational to some make complete sense to others.

The act of identity signaling, for instance, is often an attempt to affirm one's membership in a group. Doing it publicly—such as on your Instagram or Facebook profile—provides an efficient way to signal to yourself and your social community *who you are.* And as we have emphasized throughout this book, who you are is heavily determined by the norms of the groups you care about.

This psychology is used by marketers, policy makers, and leaders to cultivate a sense of identity in people they seek to influence. When done well, cultivating the right kind of identity can lead to a deeper sense of connection and, for companies, a stronger bottom line. Understanding the dynamics of social identity has allowed some organizations to corner their markets and others to encompass the globe. We believe, for example, that Apple became one of the world's largest companies not only through technical savvy but by creating in many consumers a deep sense of identification with its products. Like Molson Canadian, Apple built an identity that meets a psychological need for *optimal distinctiveness*—the feeling that you simultaneously belong and stand out from others. It's a potent cocktail.

Psychological needs can help us understand what motivates people to identify with groups. What is it that makes some groups more attractive than others or more attractive at certain points in people's lives? We will explore the role that belonging, distinctiveness, and status play in binding people to groups. Groups that fulfill one or more of these goals are going to be more appealing than groups that do not. When social identities scratch these motivational itches, people place more value on these groups and on the things and actions that symbolize their memberships.

This chapter will also dive more deeply into the ways that social identities provide potent incentives for cooperation. We will present evidence showing how people more readily cooperate and improve outcomes for everyone when they identify with their groups and adhere to cooperative social norms. This has critical implications for creating groups and organizations that function effectively.

If employees, for example, care only about personal outcomes like wages and bonuses, they will often find a way to game the system and exploit loopholes for personal gain. Petty theft by their own employees is estimated to cost companies tens of billions of dollars each year, an average of 1.4 percent of their revenue.[5] And this does not account for losses due to absenteeism and other ways in which people seek to benefit themselves at the expense of collective goods. If employees do not identify with their organizations, they will do what it takes to benefit or protect themselves personally, not necessarily what is good for their firms. Organizations operate much more effectively when people identify with them.

VALUING OTHERS

When the two of us arrived at The Ohio State University, it quickly became clear that the identity of the university community was centered on the college football team, the Buckeyes. At every home game, the campus was overrun with more than a hundred thousand fans dressed in scarlet and gray. Every bar was packed. TVs were placed in every restaurant in the city, and they all carried the game live (followed by countless hours of replays and analysis). It was a celebration of collective purpose unlike anything we had ever seen.

The year we arrived on campus, the team won their first twelve games and went on to play in the national championship game. It was clear to us that the Buckeyes knew something special about group success.

Nearly forty years earlier, the football team had started one of the most interesting traditions in college sports. According to legend, a member of the coaching staff had an idea to motivate the players.[6] After each game, the coaches would reward the best players by giving them small stickers to place on their helmets.

The logic was simple: recognizing individual success would provide a social incentive for players to work harder to stand out. The stickers would become symbols of individual achievement, and by the end of the season, star players would stroll onto the field with their helmets covered in small Ohio Buckeye symbols, not unlike military generals decorated in medals. The Buckeyes won the national championship that year, and teams around the country copied the practice of using stickers to reward excellence.

The stickers became an institution. But by 2001, the long

successful Buckeyes had returned to mediocrity. So when the team hired a new coach, Jim Tressel, he decided to mess with tradition. Rather than recognizing individual performance, Tressel changed the reward system to focus on collective success. For example, instead of giving one player a sticker for scoring a touchdown, every player on the offensive unit would get a sticker if the team scored a certain number of points. And the coaches gave every player on the team a sticker after each win.

Rewarding teamwork paid off, and the team won a national championship the next year. By encouraging the players to value collective success rather than just individual accomplishments, the coaches had managed to generate effective cooperation. By the time we arrived on campus, the Buckeyes had cemented their record as one of the most successful teams in the country.[7]

This helped explain the camaraderie in the locker room and on the field. But the benefits of shared identity extended far beyond the football field, creating a shared sense of purpose—and pride— among a much broader swath of people. We were not the first social psychologists at Ohio State to recognize the impact of this social identity on the fans. More than three decades before we arrived on campus, Robert Cialdini and his collaborators studied how people who were not part of the game nevertheless felt the warm glow of success after a victory.[8] Fans contribute little to the success of the team beyond their moral support, but they might well "bask in reflected glory" when the team triumphs.

College football games are played on Saturdays, so the researchers monitored students at seven different universities to see who showed up wearing team-supporting apparel in class on Mondays. They counted buttons, jackets, T-shirts, sweaters, and briefcases that displayed the school logo or team nickname and found that 8 percent of students wore university apparel to class that semester. On Mondays after their home team had won a game, however, this number spiked.

Visible signals of identification with the team surged on these days as students became more likely to wear school symbols to class in a show of pride. In a subsequent study, the researchers called students after each game and asked them to describe the outcome. After victories, students were more likely to use collective pronouns to describe the event, saying "we won" as opposed to "the team won." But the use of the word *we* diminished following losses. In fact, students used the term *we* when describing a victory nearly twice as often (26 percent) as they did when describing a loss (13.5 percent).

These findings suggest that people identified with their team more following a win than a loss. But were they simply sporting team-promoting garb to fit in with everyone else following a victory or was there more to it than that? Did they genuinely experience a ray of reflected glory?

To better grasp how identities influence the way people value the outcomes of others, we used functional neuroimaging to look inside New York University students' brains as their in-group succeeded. In a project led by Leor Hackel, we brought students into NYU's Center for Brain Imaging and had them play an economic game with either an in-group member (a fellow NYU student) or an out-group member (a student from Columbia University).[9] In this game, they had the chance to earn real money based on their decisions.

On half the trials, we gave them a choice between an amount of money they could take for themselves (for example, a dollar) or an amount of money they could give to the other player (for example, two dollars). In this case, people most often preferred to grab the dollar for themselves, but sometimes they felt generous enough to allow the other player to walk away with the larger sum. When students confronted these types of decisions, however, it mattered a great deal whom they were playing with.

When highly identified NYU students were playing with a fellow NYU student, they were more generous than when they were playing with a Columbia student. This pattern reversed among students who were not strongly identified with NYU. If anything, these students were slightly more generous to an out-group member. In other words, people were willing to sacrifice their own money to help out an in-group member over an out-group member—but only if they identified with the in-group.

We then analyzed patterns of neural activity. To examine how people valued others' outcomes, the study also included a number of trials in which our participants received money at no one else's expense, as well as trials in which they observed their partner (the in-group or out-group member) receiving money at no one else's expense. This allowed us to identify a small region of the brain, known as the right caudate, that was especially active when participants received a reward. Having identified this region, we looked to see whether it was also active when a member of the in-group, a fellow NYU student, received a reward—and it was! The same region that responded when they personally were given money responded to the sight of an in-group member experiencing this positive outcome. This did not happen, of course, when they watched an out-group member being rewarded.

This neuroscience approach gives us insight into whether people are genuinely basking in the reflected glory of in-group members when something good happens to them or if they, for example, are wearing the team jersey after a victory merely to fit in on campus. Our study suggests that something akin to genuine basking does occur; people who care about the in-group are not only willing to send fellow members more money than they send rival out-group members but also appear to have an intrinsic feeling of reward when fellow group members have a stroke of good fortune.

This underscores a virtue of identity: it is one of the reasons we care about the outcomes of others. The feelings of joy you get when a teammate succeeds, a colleague wins an award, or your country wins a medal at the Olympics are all evidence of identity-based value in operation.

FITTING IN

Humans have a powerful need to belong, fit in, and connect with others. The consequences of not fitting in can be severe. Loneliness, the feeling that one lacks meaningful social connection with others, is a well-known contributor to poorer mental- and physical-health outcomes. Indeed, the sociologist Robert Putnam famously declared that if someone smokes a pack of cigarettes a day and belongs to no groups, it is a statistical toss-up as to which he or she should change. Quit smoking or join a group—either will have about the same impact on your health.[10]

Joining groups is good for your health because, among other things, it satisfies core human motivations. During the COVID-19 pandemic, Dom and a group of colleagues examined how social identities embedded in people's local communities were associated with poor mental-health outcomes like stress and depression. From April to October of 2020, we observed that people who felt more connected to their communities—especially those who believed that members of their communities were rallying to support one another during the crisis—experienced less stress and depression over time.

Groups that provide a sense of belonging are often attractive to people because they satisfy this essential need. People may also find social identities more important when they are experiencing a heightened desire to belong, either chronically (some people seem to feel this need more strongly than others) or in a particular situation.

Some of our research has examined one of the consequences of this; namely, that people are more attentive to and remember fellow group members better when their need to belong is active. People often exhibit better memory for the faces of in-group compared to out-group members. For example, it is common for people to recognize faces belonging to their own racial categories more readily than faces of people of other races. This is partly why people sometimes say that members of other groups seem to look alike. To some extent, this is probably due to differences in experience. People generally spend more time, especially early in life, around others who belong to the same racial groups as themselves, and they may develop some expertise at recognizing certain types of faces.

But this is not the whole story.[11] It turns out that people are better at recognizing in-group members generally, even when people in their in-group belong to different races or when an in-group and out-group are all the same race and cannot be distinguished in that way. In several experiments, we assigned people to completely novel teams (minimal-type groups) that they had never heard of before.[12] After they joined their groups, we showed participants a series of faces of both in-group and out-group members before giving them a surprise memory test.

Generally speaking, people remember the in-group faces better than out-group faces, probably because they pay more attention to them when they are first encountered. The people in our own groups are often more relevant to us and so they get more of our concentration. However, this difference is larger for people who have a stronger need to belong. Hungry for social connection, they are more attuned than ever to fellow in-group members.

The need to belong may also influence how people value symbols and products attached to their identities. Researchers in the Netherlands conducted experiments in which they made people feel excluded, thus heightening their need to belong, before having them choose between different kinds of Dutch products.[13] Critically, some of the products were nostalgic—from brands that were popular in the nation's past. Other products were contemporary, popular only in the here and now. They found that people who had been excluded were more nostalgic, choosing brands of cookies, crackers, soup, candy, and cars with roots in the past more often than people who had not been made to feel excluded.

Meeting belongingness needs is often difficult. These challenges may be particularly acute for members of minority or marginalized groups who often get treated in ways that imply they do not fully belong. Although they might have been citizens of a country for many years or across multiple generations, members of visual minority groups are frequently asked, "Where do you come from?" or "What is your background?" as if their identity must reside elsewhere.

In a pair of experiments, Maya Guendelman and her colleagues studied how these sorts of identity threats influence food choices, speculating that people singled out as different due to their ethnic or cultural background might feel the need to work extra-hard to confirm their identity as Americans.[14] They recruited Asian Americans (with heritage from a variety of countries in Asia), who, despite being born in the United States, are often told they don't belong.

When the participants arrived in the lab, the experimenter—a White American—asked half of them if they spoke English. This might seem like an innocent query on the surface, but to many minority group members, it serves as a signal that their identity as an American is being questioned.

When they were asked about their food preferences, the Asian American participants who had been asked if they spoke English were three times more likely to say that their favorite foods were typical American fare—things like Big Macs and pizzas—than Asian Americans who had not been queried about their language. The same question about speaking English had no influence on White American participants, likely because it was not experienced as a threat to belonging by these majority group members.

In a subsequent experiment, participants were given access to a food-delivery website and asked to select a dish they wanted to eat. If they had been asked about speaking English, Asian Americans were more likely to order hot dogs, hamburgers, fried chicken, and Philly cheesesteaks over less typically American choices like sushi, pork banh mi, bibimbap, and chicken curry. Selecting the American food options was unhealthy, translating into choices that contained, on average, an extra 182 calories and 12 grams of fat compared to the food selected by Asian Americans who had not been asked about speaking English. However, choosing stereotypically American foods might have helped Asian Americans feel (or allowed them to demonstrate) a stronger sense of national belonging after it had been called into question.

THINK DIFFERENT

More than seventy-seven million people watched the 1984 Super Bowl between the Washington, DC, NFL team and the Los Angeles Raiders. The game itself has long been forgotten by everyone but the most die-hard fans, but many people still remember the striking commercial that aired during an advertising break.

In a scene from a dystopian future, row upon row of people sit transfixed as they watch Big Brother on a huge video screen. A voice drones on about the "first glorious anniversary of the Information Purification Directives." Suddenly, out of nowhere, a blond woman comes running past the passive rows of spectators. As she reaches the front, she hurls an enormous, Thor-like hammer at the screen and smashes it to smithereens. Then a voice-over message: "On January 24, Apple Computer will introduce Macintosh. And you'll see why 1984 won't be like *1984*."

In a competitive field, the famous 1984 Apple commercial was named the best Super Bowl advertising spot in the game's forty-year history, and *TV Guide* ranked it as the number-one commercial of all time. The ad marked the beginning of a revolutionary advertising sequence in which Apple positioned itself as the signature computer brand for rebels—for people who stand out as distinctive. Building on the theme, over a decade later, Apple launched its "Think Different" campaign featuring iconoclastic figures like Albert Einstein,

Martin Luther King Jr., Amelia Earhart, and Pablo Picasso. They cemented the idea that Apple was the brand for mavericks and innovators.

These commercials might seem ironic now, when Apple is one of the most ubiquitous and valuable companies on earth. It is impossible to grab coffee or groceries without noticing that you are surrounded by people using Apple products. You could be forgiven for thinking that, far from being anti-conformists or rebels, Apple users are not that different from the drones in that famous commercial: transfixed by a screen, inattentive to the world around them.

Indeed, the two of us are as likely as anyone else to be caught staring mindlessly at our iPhones as we stroll around campus. Yet we also like to maintain the image of ourselves as rebels who flout convention. How is it that Apple managed to cultivate the sense that its users "Think Different" while also turning them into one of the largest groups of consumer conformists in history? The answer is that Apple became one of the world's most successful and valuable brands, with a cultlike following, by creating an *optimally distinct identity*.

The idea of "optimal distinctiveness" was developed by one of our mentors and intellectual heroes, Marilynn Brewer.[15] She understood that the most compelling groups are often those that fulfill two basic but conflicting human motives: a need to belong and a need to be distinctive. People want to belong, but part of the power of a social identity comes from what it excludes—which helps people clarify who they are and who they are not.

As Brewer put it, we seek to be the same and different at the same time.

Picture a group of punks, or goths, or hipsters. If you're like us, you're probably imagining a few young people dressed in much the same way as one another, adorned with similar jewelry, piercings, or tattoos, listening to the same music through the same style of headphones. If you actually ran into a group like this on the street, you might be tempted to ask, *Don't you know that you all look the same?* To which they might offer the snarky reply: *No way—you're the conformist; we're expressing our individuality!* These sorts of subcultures embody optimal distinctiveness in action. Their members experience a delightful sense of *distinctiveness from the rest of society* while benefiting from a deep sense of *belonging with their own kind.* Achieving this sort of balance is one of the reasons why certain groups prove irresistible to people.

The same psychology applies to products. By purchasing certain products, you reveal to yourself—and others—who you think you are. The sort of car you drive, clothing you wear, foods you eat, and technologies you use can send signals to others. They may sometimes be signifiers of status (your level of wealth, for example), but often these choices seem to express something more about what you value and the identities you hold dear.

You might be hesitant to believe that people truly identify with a product like Apple. We were, too, so we ran a study to investigate. Dominic surveyed students at Lehigh University to learn about their most cherished identities. As one would expect, identities related to gender, race, age, and politics were common. But sure enough, a significant number of students said they were proud to be either a "Mac" or a "PC" person.

Other research has found that the appeal of optimal distinctiveness extends to charitable decisions. For instance, an analysis of over twenty-eight thousand crowdfunding campaigns found that distinctiveness was a key ingredient for success.[16] Those campaigns that stood out from traditional narratives about similar types of causes were more appealing; they attracted more financial backers and raised more money. People tend to be drawn to narratives that differentiate a cause, defining how it is special.

THE APPEAL OF UNDERDOGS

The psychological magic of optimal distinctiveness helps us understand why music fans will brag that they liked a famous band or musician "before they were big" and why people love to cheer for the underdog. By definition, underdogs are likely to lose and might seem like a bad place to align your identity, since they will leave you crying into your beer more often than not. But we have found that people who have a heightened need for distinctiveness are more likely to identify with underdogs.

When the two of us were in graduate school, we came across a newspaper article about Microsoft claiming that it was an underdog in its battle with its Silicon Valley rivals. At the time, Microsoft was one of the largest and most powerful companies in the world, the recent target of an antitrust lawsuit from the U.S. government. It seemed strange to us that such a large and powerful company would try to claim underdog status, unless executives were doing it to increase how much their employees—and their customers—identified with their company.

To find out whether underdogs help satisfy the need for optimal distinctiveness, we designed studies in collaboration with Geoff Leonardelli, a professor at the University of Toronto's business school. Toronto is the largest university in the country, and, as in large groups generally, students often complain that they are treated as if they are anonymous, not as distinctive individuals. In our studies, we exacerbated this feeling for some of our student participants, stating that the university saw them simply as a number, one among thousands, thereby heightening the student's need or desire for a distinct identity.

For other students in these studies, we affirmed that they were seen as unique individuals rather than as mere numbers. Their desire for uniqueness satisfied, these participants, we hypothesized, would not need to identify with an underdog to scratch that itch.

139

We then had everyone read about the university's men's water polo team. (We selected the water polo team because hardly anyone had heard of it, which made it easy for us to shape their impressions of the team.) We told some participants that the team was entering an upcoming championship game as an underdog; we told others that the team was the clear favorite to win.

Rationally, one might think that students would especially want to cheer on their own university's team if it was a success story and favored to win. But this was not exactly what we found. Instead, people who felt a need for distinctiveness because we, the researchers, had made them feel like mere anonymous cogs were more likely to identify with the water polo team when they were the *underdog*.

We found a similar pattern in a subsequent study in which we measured identification with two NBA teams—the New York Knicks and the Miami Heat—locked in a close playoff game. Again, the underdog team was more appealing to the folks whose need for a distinctive identity was heightened. The feeling seemed to spike when the underdogs pulled close at the end of the game and fans could taste victory.

This might be why sports stories about underdogs are eternally appealing. People want to achieve a level of optimal distinctiveness, and identifying with an underdog helps meet the balance between fitting in and standing apart. It changes the psychological value of a team that is otherwise a long shot. As a result (we think), Hollywood produces a near-endless stream of movies about underdogs.

From *Rocky* to *Hoosiers* to *Rudy* to *A League of Their Own* to *The Mighty Ducks,* the appeal of the underdog crosses sports and generations. But people want to do more than simply support underdogs or, more generally, possess optimally distinctive identities. They often want to signal these identities to the world.

SIGNALING IDENTITY

Apple recognized that its customers not only bought its products—they became brand evangelists. Can you think of something that comes with every Apple product that has absolutely no practical function?

If you are an Apple enthusiast, you know that every major Apple product comes with a small white sticker depicting the famous bitten-apple logo. The sticker serves no purpose; it is not even meant to go on the product itself. The function is entirely social. You can place the Apple sticker on your bike, car window, or suitcase to signal to others at work, school, and in transit that they are in the presence of a Mac person.

Apple also built this signaling sensibility into its products. For example, the Apple logo on the lid of every laptop faces down and away from the person who owns it when the lid is closed. This might seem like a mistake, but it's not. Once the computer is opened, the logo faces the right way up to *other people* across the room. It is an identity signal to others, not the self.

Economists have found that people will pay large amounts of money to signal a distinctive identity. One of the most interesting—and expensive—ways that people signal identity is through the vehicles they drive.[17] Environmentalism has become an important part of some people's identities, which has created a market for electric or hybrid cars that offer better mileage and are less harmful to the environment. For a long time, perhaps the most distinctive hybrid car was the Toyota Prius. One of the first widely produced electric cars on the market, it had a visually unique style that was easily noticed by other environmentally conscious bystanders.

Economists observed that people were willing to pay more for a Prius than for a comparable hybrid car, the Honda Civic. Both cars offered roughly the same environmental benefits in terms of mileage and emissions, but the Honda Civic did so in a more subtle fashion. The Civic is a popular model of car and had been around for years before Honda decided to make a hybrid version. There were thousands of nonhybrid but very similar-looking Honda Civics on the road, making it difficult for your coworker or neighbor to realize that you were driving a hybrid. This was in stark contrast to the visually unusual Prius, which clearly signaled your environmental credentials to everyone in your social network.

This distinctiveness added value. People were willing to spend as much as $4,200 more at the time to drive the Prius. At a purely pragmatic level, this is irrational. Surely environmentalists should care more about the actual impact of a car on the environment than on their ability to signal that impact to others. However, this is not how identity works. People want to do multiple things at the same time—live out their beliefs and values while also maximizing their belonging and their distinctiveness. Driving the more obvious hybrid car allowed them to achieve this balance. Given the relatively high price tag of these cars, it might also have helped people satisfy another psychological need—the need for status.

STATUS NEEDS

On March 12, 2019, news broke that actresses Lori Loughlin and Felicity Huffman had been arrested in a massive college-bribery scandal.[18] Operation Varsity Blues alleged that thirty-three parents of college applicants had collectively paid more than twenty-five million dollars to fraudulently increase their kids' test scores or bribe university administrators. These parents were allegedly willing to break the law to give their kids a leg up in the admissions process at prestigious universities like Stanford, Yale, Northwestern, UC Berkeley, UCLA, and USC. The case was the largest of its kind to be prosecuted by the U.S. Justice Department.

The national media covered this story because it involved bad behavior by celebrities and it exposed serious corruption within the higher-education system. But at the heart of the crime were anxious and wealthy parents seeking an edge in the hypercompetitive market for college admissions.

A good education is a key to future opportunity and earnings, and tuition—especially in the United States—is often pricey. But is it worth spending hundreds of thousands more (let alone risking a prison sentence) to buy your kid an education at a slightly more prestigious school than they might otherwise attend?

Most economists would probably say no. The benefits of college are largely accrued by lower-socioeconomic-class students, and there is little difference in the actual quality of education between the more prestigious University of Southern California and the marginally less prestigious University of California, Irvine. Motivated students are just as likely to flourish at a good state school as they are at a plush private university. This is an important point that is often overlooked in reputations and rating systems. The goal of an educational institution is presumably to educate people and improve their lives, yet rankings often include factors like how hard it is to get admitted, the financial resources of the institution, and how much money the alumni give back. Critically, these metrics have recently been changing to pay more attention to student outcomes, like graduation rates, and how well a university contributes to social mobility for less advantaged students.

But rankings matter to people, as do perceptions of relative status. This helps explain why people are willing to mortgage their houses or break the law to get their kids into a marginally more prestigious university. Higher-ranked schools provide a potent social-identity boost for both students and parents.

We are not suggesting that a prestigious university pedigree doesn't confer real benefits. In addition to a wonderful opportunity to learn, these schools help determine job prospects and romantic and life partners. Students gain access to valuable social networks they may remain in for the rest of their lives. But many of these benefits are due as much to the identity their graduates now hold as they are to the gains in skills and knowledge that are fundamental to a university education.

In the landscape of higher education, membership in the Ivy League represents elite status. But there are differences in status even among those Ivy League universities. For instance, one survey found that while 41 percent of people realize that Harvard is an Ivy, less than 2 percent know that the University of Pennsylvania belongs to the same category.[19]

To outsiders, this may seem trivial, but these subtle differences in status are psychologically real to the people involved. Indeed, because their status is less well recognized, Penn students are more eager to point out their credentials to others to avoid any confusion. When Penn and Harvard students are asked to describe their university to others, Penn students are more likely to mention that they attend an Ivy League school, even in private correspondence. Harvard students don't feel as much need to mention it; people already know they have a high-status social identity.

The same psychology of identity plays out on university websites and even professors' e-mails. After all, professors are hardly immune from the same psychological needs as their students. One analysis found that lower-ranked universities were more likely to mention the word *university* on their websites than their more prestigious counterparts.[20] Departments with lower rankings were also more likely to list the credentials of their faculty. And professors did the same. As a result, faculty with more publications or citations were less likely to display symbols of personal success in their e-mail signatures.

Attempts to claim and signal a high-status social identity are part of a psychological phenomenon known as symbolic self-completion.[21] Most people need the acknowledgment of others to feel that they achieved a desired identity. When symbols of your success are recognized and affirmed by others, it reassures you that you have attained that identity in the eyes of your peers and of society. This is true not only for academic credentials but for any aspect of life in which people seek to excel, whether in their profession, their hobbies, or even their relationships. Why else is there such a market for WORLD'S BEST GRANDPA T-shirts and #1 MOM mugs?

We have noticed a tendency both on social media and offline for people to diminish and even make fun of identity signaling. Sometimes disparaged as "virtue signaling" or "showing off," the implication is that displays of identity are self-promoting or disingenuous. And certainly they can be. But signaling identities is also a vital part of the way that people navigate the social world. It is how people establish standing and how fellow members of valued groups find one another.

FINDING EACH OTHER

When humans collaborate, we are capable of extraordinary things. We build cathedrals, create universities, run multinational corporations, and cohere in nation-states. We build Mars rovers and land on the moon. We become greater than the sum of our parts. There's more to these enterprises than shared identity, of course. But identity helps people overcome hurdles to successful collaboration by making cooperation much easier.

Whenever people choose to work together, it is an act of trust. Deciding to write this book together, we trusted that each of us would uphold his end of the bargain, contributing about equally to the long hours of writing, rewriting, and more rewriting! When we signed with our agent, we trusted that he would do his utmost to find us a publisher (thanks, Jim!). And when we contracted with Little, Brown Spark, we trusted that they would do a good job editing and selling our book. They, in turn, trusted that we would write a decent book under the deadline. The fact that you are reading this book means that all these small acts of trust worked out.

There are multiple ways to decide whether you can trust someone. Establishing long relationships in which people learn about each other is one way. Legal contracts are another. And shared identities are a third. We have seen (especially in chapter 1) that when people take on a social identity, it induces a shift in motivation, and they become interested in outcomes beyond their own individual self-interest. Selfish individuals, ordinarily focused quite exclusively on their own outcomes, start to contribute as much to collective goods as pro-social people, who normally care more about other people's outcomes.

But this shift in motivation is not sufficient to produce trust. It's not enough that you care about fellow in-group members and would like to see them thrive. To really trust them and believe that they are likewise interested in your success, you need to believe that they are similarly motivated to do good by your common group membership. In other words, knowledge of identity needs to be *shared* to unlock the full potential for cooperation.

To illustrate the importance of sharing knowledge of an identity, imagine that you're playing something known as the "trust game." In every round of this game, you are given a sum of money—let's say ten dollars—and have to decide how much of it to invest with a partner. The amount that you choose to invest will be sent to your partner and will be multiplied by some amount—let's say three. So if you decide to invest the full amount and send across all ten dollars, it will multiply and your partner will receive thirty dollars. Your partner then gets to decide how much to send back to you. If that person is completely fair and sends back half of what he or she received, you will each walk away with fifteen dollars, one and a half times your original allotment, and three times what you started with collectively. Both of you do well if there is enough trust.

Now imagine that on some rounds your partner is an in-group

member and on other rounds your partner belongs to an out-group. How much would you choose to invest with each type of partner? If you're like most people, you will invest more money with an in-group than an out-group partner because you trust an in-group member more; that is, you expect that you will get more money back from that person.

But now imagine that while *you* know that you and your fellow in-group member share an identity, *your partner* is unaware of your common bond. He or she is blind to who you are! What would you do now?

Experiments that manipulate exactly this find that while people still have plenty of positive feelings toward fellow in-group members, they don't trust them more than out-group members when their own identity is not visible.[22] Knowing that an in-group member is aware that the two of you belong to the same group is the key to unlocking cooperation.

The critical importance of knowing about shared identities helps explain why people take such pains to signal their group memberships to others. Catholics wear crucifixes; liberals, conservatives, environmentalists, runners, hunters, advocates, and activists of all kinds affix bumper stickers to their cars. And people spent roughly $26.47 billion on licensed sports apparel in 2018. These and many other symbols are signs of group pride, and they play the crucial role of signaling your allegiances and identities to others.

Growing up in Canada, we were told to sew our national flag to our backpacks when we traveled abroad. As teenagers let loose in Europe (Jay in Italy, Dom in France) we met Canadian women who recognized these symbols of shared identity and were delighted to find a fellow in-group member so far from home. We had traveled to these other countries to experience new things and meet different kinds of people, but by signaling our national identity in a conspicuous way, we found and momentarily enjoyed the company of fellow in-group members among strangers.

Toshio Yamagishi, a social psychologist who initiated research on many of these issues, described social identities as "containers of generalized reciprocity."[23] What he meant was that when we share an identity with people it helps us to trust them even without knowing anything else about them. We trust that our fellow in-group members have undergone the same motivational shift that we have and are now oriented toward our collective interests.

This is how social identities allow people to establish trust with a much broader array of people than they can possibly know directly or enter into legal contracts with. It vastly expands our possibilities for connection and cooperation. Unfortunately, however, the value we place on our in-groups sometimes has a negative side. In the next chapter, we will delve into how group dynamics contribute to prejudice and discrimination—and what can be done about it.

CHAPTER 6

OVERCOMING BIAS

"This is 911, what's your emergency?" the operator asked.

"I have two gentlemen in my café who are refusing to make a purchase or leave," Holly Hylton replied.

Hylton, the on-duty manager at Starbucks in Center City, Philadelphia, made this call on the afternoon of April 12, 2018, setting in motion a cascade of events that would result in international headlines, trigger outrage across the country, and unleash demands for a boycott. Ultimately, it caused Starbucks executives to temporarily shut down nearly eight thousand stores across the United States.[1]

The gentlemen in question—two young Black men—had entered the café minutes earlier and were quietly waiting for a friend. They had not yet purchased anything and when they asked to use the restroom, they were refused access.

While this might not seem terribly unusual for many business establishments, it was outside the norm for Starbucks, which is known for allowing people to use their bathrooms. When former New York City mayor Michael Bloomberg was asked by a reporter why the city does not have more public bathrooms, he quipped, "There's enough Starbucks that'll let you use the bathroom."[2]

Alas, this courtesy didn't seem to apply to everyone.

Police officers arrived at the Starbucks and arrested the two men for trespassing despite the protests of patrons who argued that the men had not done anything wrong. The episode was caught on video and went viral.[3] People around the world saw six police officers handcuffing and removing the two men from the café while another patron (a White man) pleaded with the police to explain what they had done.

Eventually the two men were released without charges, and the Philadelphia police, as well as the city, apologized in the face of massive public outrage.

The Starbucks Corporation quickly entered damage-control mode. Hylton left her job, and a few weeks later, Starbucks announced that they would close thousands of their cafés in the United States and other nations to provide their employees with training "to address implicit bias, promote conscious inclusion, and ensure everyone inside a Starbucks store feels safe and welcome."[4]

The company's actions reflected, at that point, the largest-scale and highest-profile implementation of training based on the increasingly hot concept of implicit bias. Suddenly, everyone was talking about it. But what is implicit bias, exactly? And what strategies are effective in reducing bias?

THE ROOTS OF BIAS

Before the U.S. Congress confirms a new president's nominees for the cabinet, senators from both parties subject them to a grilling. During the hearing for Merrick Garland, President Joe Biden's choice for attorney general, Senator John Kennedy threw him a curveball. "I want to ask you about the concept of implicit bias," the Republican from Louisiana said. "Does that mean I'm a racist, no matter what I do or what I think? I'm a racist, but I don't know I'm a racist?"

Though his queries might have been intended to discomfit

Garland or trip him up, they reflect the sorts of questions that many people have about what it means to be prejudiced and what the distinctions are between different forms of bias.

Over the past several decades, scientists have developed a variety of tests to measure implicit or unconscious biases, capturing the preferences that people have toward some groups over others that they are not necessarily fully aware of.[5] These tests are designed to measure the feelings and associations that rapidly and automatically come to mind when people encounter members of different groups. In fact, they can be used to assess quick reactions to all sorts of things, not just social groups—types of food, addictive substances, animals, and so on.

Icebergs are often used as a metaphor for the human mind. While your conscious experiences appear to dominate your mental life, they are actually just the tip of a much larger structure, most of which lies hidden beneath the surface. Many functions of the mind operate automatically or outside your awareness, and by the time you become consciously aware of things, a significant amount of information processing has already occurred.

For some things, this is obvious. Your brain regulates your breathing and digestion without you consciously giving it a second thought. What is sometimes more surprising to people is that a great deal of unconscious, uncontrolled, and often very quick processing also takes place as you make sense of other people.

Explicit biases are ones that people talk about. If someone says or indicates on a survey that she doesn't like millennials or Canadians, she is expressing a clear and presumably unashamed prejudice. These sorts of expressions tend to reflect the social norms in an environment—people are usually willing to say only what they think is acceptable. Measuring implicit bias requires more subtle tests.

On many of these tests, participants are presented with images at rapid speed of people belonging to different groups. They might be faces of men and women, Christians and Muslims, or Black or White people. You will be asked to respond to the images, and based on the pattern of your responses—how quickly you react or the types of errors you make—researchers are able to estimate your automatic preferences for different groups. For example, during a task that we have used a lot (known as "evaluative priming"), you will see a male or a female face for a few milliseconds followed by an image of something that most people find positive or negative—a cute puppy or a hairy spider, perhaps. Your task is simply to press one key on the computer if what you are looking at is something you like and another key if it is something you dislike. It turns out that the face you see before you respond to the puppy or spider can affect how quickly you classify that image as positive or negative. If you have more negative implicit reactions to male faces than female ones, for example, you will be a bit faster to say that the spider is bad after you see a man's face than after you see a woman's face. You will also be slower to say that the puppy is good after seeing a man's face.

You can try another version of an implicit bias measure, the Implicit Association Test (or IAT) yourself at Project Implicit, based at Harvard University. Having administered millions of these kinds of tests, scientists have found that the vast majority of people show some degree of implicit bias, favoring their own ethnic, national, political, or religious groups over corresponding out-groups. Of course, not everyone shows the same degree or type of bias. Many people are troubled to learn that they harbor these racial, gender, or other biases because they believe in the value of treating people equally.

Even very young children have taken variants of these tests and exhibit preferences for members of their own race, leading *Newsweek* magazine to run a provocative cover asking, "Is Your Baby Racist?"[6] Mahzarin Banaji and Anthony Greenwald, two of the scientists who developed the IAT, refer to the subtle biases possessed by otherwise good people as a "blind spot."

So what does this mean? Are humans somehow hardwired to be

racist? And if not, where do these biases come from and why do they persist even among people who think of themselves as unprejudiced and egalitarian?

If humans were truly hardwired for racism, we would expect that our species had evolved in environments where it was adaptive to differentiate among and discriminate against people from other races. Yet from everything we know about human evolution, this is unlikely.

Evolutionary psychologist Leda Cosmides and her colleagues argue they have ruled out "the hypothesis that the brain mechanisms that cause race encoding evolved for that purpose."[7] What this means is that while our brains can and do judge people on the basis of their race, we have not evolved any special neural function just for this purpose. Cosmides and her team suggest that natural selection may well have favored brain machinery that automatically registers gender and age because our ancestors inhabited a social world in which knowing other people's genders and life stages enabled them to make a variety of useful judgments about them: Who was a potential mate? Who, young or very old, was likely to need extra help?

But, Cosmides and her colleagues argue, race is different.

First, they note that "geneticists have shown that humanity is not divided into distinct racial types." Second, they provide a common-sense reason why racism would not be hardwired into our species: our ancestors were hunter-gatherers who lived in small groups and traveled primarily by foot. This meant that typical humans would almost never have encountered people from groups genetically distant enough to qualify as belonging to a different race. If they never (or very rarely) encountered people with different skin tones or facial features, there could have been no evolutionary advantage for racism.

Then why is racism such a common feature of contemporary life? One reason, they argue, is that paying close attention to race and dividing the world up on that basis is a side effect of neural machinery that was carved by natural selection to identify in-groups and track coalitions. Our ancestors lived in bands that often came into contact with other local bands. Their need to work with in-group members and defend against out-groups might have selected for people who were skilled at making "us-versus-them" distinctions and who defended the group against hostile outsiders (who tended to look a lot like them).

People also formed coalitions within bands. To grab political power or gain access to scarce food and other resources, it helped to work together. The ability to detect and identify with shifting alliances is thought to exist in every culture on earth.[8] It is a deeply human trait. We see it happening, for instance, in the minimal-group experiments discussed in chapter 1, when merely being assigned to an arbitrary category caused people to immediately form a social identity and discriminate in favor of it. Similar patterns of coalitional behavior have also been observed in other primates, our close genetic cousins, although humans might be alone among primates in our willingness to help in-group members even if they are anonymous. We are a truly groupish species.

But our evolutionary heritage also comes with a tendency for us to form and protect hierarchies that put some people and groups at the top and others at the bottom. This helps to explain why, having divided the world into categories like race, religion, and nationality, humans have the abhorrent tendency to create and defend systems of oppression.

The drive to defend group hierarchies is what political psychologist Jim Sidanius described as an orientation toward social dominance.[9] This tendency provides the psychological foundation for much of the racism that exists around the globe. From this perspective, racism is not grounded in genetic racial differences, despite what White supremacists would have you believe. Instead, it is built on mental tendencies to carve the world into groups and defend inequitable systems and power disparities.

LONG HISTORIES

Racist and other oppressive social systems have long histories. Hardly unique in this sense, racism has plagued the United States since 1619, when a ship carrying people enslaved from the African continent arrived in the colony of Virginia. America did not declare independence from Britain until 1776, but at that point slavery was already embedded within institutions and accounted for much of the nation's early wealth.

The residue of this dark history is still evident today.

It was evident in the summer of 2014 in Ferguson, Missouri, when a young Black man, Michael Brown, was shot and killed by a police officer. It was evident in New York City that same year when Eric Garner, a middle-aged Black man, was killed by an NYPD officer using a prohibited choke hold. And it was evident in the spring of 2020 when Breonna Taylor was shot by police while sleeping in her Louisville apartment and when, shortly thereafter, a Minneapolis officer killed George Floyd by kneeling on his neck for nine minutes and twenty-nine seconds.

Police killings of Black and other people of color are shockingly common in the United States. Exactly the same words with which sociologist Gunnar Myrdal described racial disparities in justice in the early 1940s can be used, unedited, today. He wrote, "The police often assume the duty not only of arresting but also of sentencing and punishing the culprit."[10] But what makes these killings resemble the past is also the impunity of many of the police officers involved. In the cases of Michael Brown, Eric Garner, and Breonna Taylor, public prosecutors brought potential charges to a grand jury, and the jury declined to indict the officers. These were not decisions to find the officers not guilty; they were decisions not to even hold a trial.

The way people evaluate and react to each other in the present is the result of multiple influences operating on different time scales. It is like a complex tone—or sound wave—made up of a set of constituent frequencies. Some of these frequencies oscillate rapidly, on the scale of days, minutes, or seconds. Some are slower, operating over years or decades as a person is socialized, develops, and has life experiences. Others may be slower still, operating over generations, carrying undertones from the deep past into the present.

In recent years, social scientists have started to study the effects of slavery on current-day outcomes. For example, economists have found that locations in the United States where more people were enslaved in the 1800s tend to have higher levels of economic inequality and remain economically underdeveloped today.[11] We and other researchers have similarly found that a history of slavery in certain parts of the United States relates to attitudes and biases in the present.[12] Based on data from about 1.8 million White participants who took an online Black/White IAT on the Project Implicit website between 2001 and 2013, we looked at relationships between current-day levels of bias in particular locations and what had happened in those places in the past. We observed that levels of implicit bias today were greater in former slaveholding states.

When we took a deeper look, we found higher implicit bias among people who live in Southern counties today that in the year 1860 had relatively more enslaved Black people living there. In other words, the ratio of enslaved Black people to the White population in a county in 1860 predicted White residents having more implicit racial bias in that county today. It predicted higher explicit bias as well.

It is, in part, the stability of the social environment that holds racist identities and attitudes in place.[13] Whether people are aware of it or not, symbolic and structural features of environments, from the symbolism of the Confederate flag to separation of racial groups in segregated neighborhoods and schools, perpetuate old patterns. Biases are persistent in large part because people live in a world that has yet to fully abolish old legacies of structural and institutional discrimination.

Many people are becoming more aware of the impact of these

systemic features of racism. As we were writing this book, protesters around the world were dismantling symbols of oppressive history. In the United States, nearly one hundred Confederate monuments were removed in 2020; in Richmond, Virginia, people threw a statue of Christopher Columbus into a lake.[14] In Antwerp, Belgium, people set fire to a statue of King Leopold II.

These events reflect an effort to restructure environments to produce different attitudes and norms. By recognizing the impact of past oppression and dismantling its symbols, people hope to create more inclusive identities for future generations. Charting a new course for the future often requires grappling with the past. And how to do this effectively is not always straightforward.

Research linking current-day attitudes to historical circumstances makes it clear that there are unlikely to be any quick fixes when it comes to problems of racism and other forms of bias. Yet understanding the psychological roots of bias can shed light on potential pathways for reducing it. The psychology of social identity can be used to bridge divides rather than create them. Given our species' capacity to form identities around new groups, finding different ways of dividing up the social world can have positive effects. Indeed, creating new identities can reshape the automatic mind.

WIRED FOR SOCIAL IDENTITY

The two of us became interested in how identities affect implicit bias when we were sharing an office as graduate students. Around that time, there was a sense among many researchers that implicit racial biases were probably inevitable. It was assumed that after people were exposed for years to all of their society's stereotypes and prejudices, negative associations with marginalized groups would become deeply entrenched in their minds. Scholars found it difficult to reduce implicit bias in the lab, and measures of implicit bias were often quite disconnected from the explicit attitudes and values that people expressed in surveys or in public.

But we were curious—just how sticky were implicit racial biases? Could we override these biases by getting people to adopt a new, more inclusive identity?

To find out, we drove about a hundred and sixty miles from our office in Toronto to Kingston, Ontario, where Queen's University had just built a new center for neuroscience and we were able to book the whole facility for large blocks of time. Wil Cunningham, our mentor, had to rent a car because his 1995 green Ford Escort did not have enough room for all of us (and none of us students could afford a car at that point). We lived out of a cheap hotel and spent our summer days in the basement of the brain center running participants through the functional neuroimaging scanner.

In previous brain-imaging studies, researchers had found that White participants consistently showed a pattern of racial bias in their neural responses when they saw people from different races. People who exhibited stronger implicit associations between *Black* and *bad* (as well as *White* and *good*) on the IAT showed greater blood flow in a small, almond-shaped region of the brain known as the amygdala.[15] This relationship between implicit bias and brain activity was especially strong when subjects were presented with people's faces for only a few milliseconds—less than the blink of an eye! This implied that the pattern of racial bias was happening very quickly in the brain and without their conscious awareness.[16]

At the time, the amygdala was widely believed to be centrally involved in the processing of negative emotions. However, our lab, as well as a few others, had begun to accumulate evidence that this brain area was perhaps better understood as reacting to highly relevant or important stimuli, from erotic images to famous celebrities. It seemed to be signaling something like *Pay attention to this!* Often, these signals were for negative or unfamiliar things, like out-groups. But positive things can be highly relevant and important too, especially when they are connected to our sense of identity.

The question we asked that summer was what would happen to brain activity in this region if participants felt a sense of shared identity with people of different races. This happens all the time at school, at work, and in sports, when people find themselves sharing groups and goals with people from any number of different backgrounds and ethnicities. We suspected that sharing a common identity might be enough to change the typically observed patterns of racial bias. To see if this was the case, we assigned our participants, all of whom were White, to a mixed-race team. Just as in the minimal-group studies, we created these teams by flipping a coin.[17]

People came to the study one at a time; we took each person's photo and uploaded it to a computer. In the first phase, the participants were told they would join one of two teams, the Leopards or the Tigers. For the next few minutes, they memorized photos of twelve people who were members of their in-group and photos of twelve other people who were members of the out-group. They also saw their own photo in the mix to help them identify with their team. Critically, the photos were racially diverse; half the members of each team were White and half were Black.

The people in our study were now part of a mixed-race team, although they would never have a chance to meet or learn more about one another. They merely looked at the other team members' faces. Would this be enough to change how their brains encoded in-group and out-group members, or would they still exhibit the standard patterns of racial bias that are so pervasive in society?

Once they were in the brain scanner (picture an appliance the size of a small kitchen with a tunnel just large enough to fit an adult), the subjects could see and react to images projected onto a mirror a few inches in front of their eyes. As they lay on their backs, they saw a random series of faces, each one an in-group or an out-group member, for two seconds at a time. When they saw a face, participants made a simple response using a button box they were holding. Sometimes they were asked to indicate whether a face belonged to an in-group or an out-group member, other times whether it was a Black or White person.

This type of research is slow and quite expensive, so it took us several trips to Kingston and many days in the imaging center to collect all the data we needed. Once the study was finished, Professor Cunningham warned us not to get too excited about any preliminary results. Although he was normally the most enthusiastic faculty member we knew—brimming with big ideas and excited about new data—he sternly reminded us that we would need many more weeks to confirm the findings and interpret them properly. But as we leaned over his computer in our lab back in Toronto, our first glimpse of the results hinted that a radical shift had occurred in our participants moments after they joined a mixed-race team.

Each subject's brain responses reflected the person's new identity as a Leopard or a Tiger. Unlike in previous studies, we could see that our participants were not responding to the race of the faces but to their new group identity—their team. More specifically, we observed greater activity in our participants' amygdalae when they saw members of their in-group compared to members of the out-group—and, critically, this occurred regardless of their teammates' race. Now that another identity was central to the situation, race had little to no bearing on how their brains responded to the faces.

The greater activation we observed in the amygdalae when people saw in-group faces was consistent with our findings that this region responds to things that are highly relevant to people. Their brains reflected a newfound affinity for the in-group that was most salient to them at that moment. Far from being wired for racism, our brains are, if anything, *wired for social identity.*

We then examined other measures of bias using data we collected during the study. We had asked people to report how much they liked or disliked each of the faces they saw. Mirroring their brain activity, people reported liking members of their in-group significantly more than members of the out-group. And again, this was unrelated to race. People liked both the Black and White members of their team equally and they felt fairly neutral toward the out-group.

Over the past fifteen years, in studies with larger samples at other universities and in another country, we have repeatedly found similar results.[18] For instance, in a study we ran with developmental neuroscientists João Guassi Moreira and Eva Telzer, we observed similar patterns of in-group bias in brain responses and behavior in children as young as eight years old.[19] The effects grew larger with age. By middle adolescence, there was a very strong relationship between their amygdalae activity toward in-group members and the level of in-group favoritism they reported to our research team.

Even on implicit measures, people consistently express a preference for members of newly created in-groups compared to out-groups. And seemingly trivial new identities like these are able to override the typical patterns of racial bias that show up time and again. Other labs have noted similar results.[20] Whether scientists are studying novel teams like the Leopards and Tigers, college rivalries, or political identities, these sorts of allegiances are consistently able to override implicit racial biases. This underscores the power of identity.

In one of the largest studies, involving more than seventeen thousand participants, Calvin Lai and his colleagues tested seventeen different possible strategies for reducing implicit racial bias.[21] They found that shifting group boundaries to form new identities, as we had done, was one of the most effective. Mere membership in a group is sufficient to change one's identity and preferences. It can bridge old divides, like race, while creating new ones. In this way, identity is, of course, a mixed blessing—it can bring you closer to a stranger but also push you away from a neighbor.

This is not to say we expected that the new and artificial identities we created in the lab would forever override racial biases or necessarily do so even once participants left the brain-imaging facility. We have seen that racial and other biases are far too robust for that, grounded as they are in persistently inequitable social systems.

In their study of bias-reduction strategies, Lai and colleagues found that even successful interventions tended not to have very long-lasting effects. In the case of novel identities, the power of a new team to override implicit and automatic racist reactions seemed to dissipate within twenty-four hours. Once people are back among the structures and patterns of their regular worlds, race-based divisions reassert themselves. However, these lab-based studies provide a powerful proof of concept, showing how creating identities might provide solutions to bias—if only we can sustain them.

The next question is whether one can take these sorts of findings from the lab and apply them to the real world, where it matters. Can building more robust real-world identities have enduring benefits for intergroup harmony? Luckily for us, other scholars have investigated just that.

THE SOCCER CURE

In 2014, ISIS, a jihadist group that follows a fundamentalist variant of Sunni Islam, committed genocide against religious minorities in northern Iraq. The terrorist group became known and feared around the world for videos of executions, often by beheading their victims. By June, they had declared themselves a worldwide caliphate and began referring to themselves as the Islamic State.

As the ISIS campaign advanced, a great many people were forced to flee their homes and live in refugee camps. Eventually, after their cities were liberated following the Battle of Mosul in 2016, refugees were able to trickle back to their homes. Many found their neighborhoods destroyed. What ISIS and their combatants had not looted, they had torched on the way out. They left a path of devastation in their wake.

These events decimated social cohesion in the region and were especially damaging to relations between Muslims and Christians. According to a sample of 476 Christians, 46 percent found their homes looted and 36 percent returned to find their homes destroyed. Four percent also reported family members missing or killed.

Christians felt deeply betrayed by the Sunnis, whom they often viewed as collaborators with ISIS. And most Muslims now felt uncomfortable in Christian areas. It was a time of incredible tension.

In the face of this tragedy and chaos, Salma Mousa, a then PhD student at Stanford University, wanted to study whether meaningful contact between members of these groups could begin to rebuild tolerance.[22] Despite the vast differences between these religious groups, they did have something in common: a passion for soccer. Working with local partners, she set up four soccer leagues to see if she could create positive contact and thereby provide a foundation for social cohesion in the aftermath of violence and devastation.

Team sports, like soccer, provide many of the keys for effective identity building: cooperation, a common goal, and roughly equal power among members. Leveraging the social power of team sports and the universal popularity of soccer, Salma recruited fifty-one amateur Christian teams and invited them to join a league in Ankawa and Qaraqosh.

But there was a catch.

Like much of life in these cities, amateur sports were largely segregated by religion. But Salma made each team agree to add three or four new players to its squad—players who might or might not be Christian. Plenty of eyebrows were raised. Some coaches threatened to walk away from the league.

Despite their initial protests, however, all the teams eventually agreed to these conditions. This increased the size of each team by several players. Half the teams received additional Christian players and the other half received Muslim players.

The average player was twenty-four years old, unmarried,

unemployed, with a high-school degree and a household income of roughly five hundred dollars per month. Initial surveys also revealed that the average Christian player had no Muslim friends, believed Muslims were cursed, and would not consider selling land to Muslims. But, more hopefully, the Christians also believed that Iraqis should treat one another as Iraqis first.

With the blessing of religious leaders, Mousa and her team handed out uniforms and started the league. The teams played together for two months either before or after the scorching summer months when temperatures in Iraq can reach 115 degrees.

What happened? Did this ambitious experiment cool the temperature between Christians and Muslims or was it no better than spending the summer in a traditional league? Or did things get even worse as people were forced into contact with members of a distrusted out-group?

The results were striking, and yet they were consistent with what we found in the laboratory in North America. At the end of the season, Christian players on mixed-religion teams were more willing to train with Muslims in the future, vote for a Muslim to win a sportsmanship prize, and sign up for a mixed-religion team the next season. By sharing a group identity and working together, they were able to bridge what had seemed like an impossible divide.

Mousa's study also found that team success amplified these effects. As anyone who has ever played with a championship team can tell you, success can forge an especially strong sense of shared identity, and connections between teammates can last for years. For Christian players on more successful mixed-religion teams, the warm glow of winning spilled over into their treatment of other Muslims, people who were not on their team. Three months later, they were more likely to visit a restaurant in a Muslim city and attend another mixed-religion social event.

These positive behaviors were less common among Christians who played on all-Christian teams. Cooperating with members of religious out-groups as teammates in possession of a common identity was far better for tolerance than competing against them.

This study seems remarkable even to us. That soccer identities can start to help overcome the fallout from religious genocide is hard to fathom. But in many ways, team sports are the perfect antidote to intergroup conflict. When a diverse group of people work together and adopt an identity, they develop camaraderie that, under the right conditions, extends to how they feel about each others' groups more broadly.

A sense of shared identity can extend beyond the field to fans sitting in the stands or watching at home. When Mohamed Salah, a Muslim soccer player, joined the Liverpool football club in Britain, it had a profound effect on fans. Salma Mousa and her colleagues analyzed hate-crime reports and over fifteen million tweets from soccer fans.[23] They observed that hate crimes in the Liverpool area dropped by 16 percent and that anti-Muslim tweets dropped by nearly half among Liverpool fans compared to fans from other clubs.

The lessons are hopeful ones: sharing a common identity can make people more tolerant of teammates and fellow in-group members from different ethnic and religious backgrounds. Yet in many places, there are powerful institutional and structural barriers to sustaining these sorts of connections.

INSTITUTIONAL BIASES

People are growing more aware that biases—whether in the form of racism, sexism, homophobia, or dis-ableism, to name a few—are not just in the heads of individuals. This is not only a psychological issue that can be resolved by changing hearts, minds, or social identities. Bias is also baked into our institutions, organizations, and social structures. Bias is a feature in the setup of many of our political, financial, corporate, justice, health, and other systems.

When we talk about "institutional bias," we find it helpful to distinguish between two ways that bias can manifest within institutions and organizations. One occurs when people employed by important institutions make biased decisions in the course of their work. This might be because they possess explicit prejudice or it might be because they are susceptible to the sorts of implicit biases we have talked about.

For example, people who work on the front lines of important institutions—police officers, doctors and nurses, judges, admissions officers and faculty at universities, mortgage brokers, and real estate agents—hold significant power within their domains. They make choices daily that affect people's lives. If these individuals are biased as they enact the power of their institutions, it matters. In an earlier chapter, we talked about a study of police traffic stops that found that Black and Hispanic drivers were more likely to be stopped and searched by officers than White drivers were.[24] We know that these differences were due to bias because they were larger during daylight hours, when officers were able to see the race of the drivers more easily than at night. Further, although Black drivers were less likely to be in possession of illegal materials than White drivers were, Black drivers were searched at higher rates, which resulted in more arrests.'

Similarly, judges often apply harsher sentences to Black suspects. Sexist professors are less likely to respond to e-mail inquiries from female students or might do so more rudely. And prejudiced doctors might provide worse medical care to members of minority communities. In some cases, these decisions are life-and-death.

But a second form of institutional bias is less psychological and more structural. These biases are built right into the policies, procedures, and rules by which organizations operate. They are intrinsic to the way things work and are not dependent on whether individuals are or are not biased themselves. They happen anyway because the disparate outcomes that they cause lie outside of individuals' discretion and control. Institutional biases like this are often legacies of the past that, due to the inertia that is part of many organizations, technologies, and social systems, have never been changed. Perhaps they have never even been questioned.

A fascinating analysis by *Consumer Reports* illustrated how biases built into safety testing have resulted in significantly more automobile injuries and deaths for women than men.[25] In the United States, female drivers and front passengers are about 17 percent more likely to be killed in a car accident than males, and women are 73 percent more likely to be seriously injured in a crash. Why?

The safety features on cars, which have advanced significantly over time, are based largely on the results of crash-testing. These tests are performed almost exclusively with male crash-test dummies—more specifically, with dummies modeled on a typical American male body from the 1970s: 171 pounds and 5 feet, 9 inches tall. It turns out that female and male bodies are sufficiently different that designing safety features to maximize male safety results in fatal gender disparities on the road.

When *Consumer Reports* spoke to industry experts, they heard various explanations: "Some say that developing new dummies and tests is unnecessary or too expensive, or would take too much time." It is not necessary for anyone involved to be overtly sexist (though some might be); all it takes is an aversion toward changing the status quo. Thus, a decision made by engineers in the 1970s about how to conduct safety tests continues to threaten the lives of millions of women today.

This is one reason why having women and other underrepresented groups at executive levels in companies is important. As of June 2019, Ford had the most female executives of all the large car manufacturers, with about 27 percent of vice president and above positions held by women. If there were more women in senior management at major automakers, we suspect that this sort of safety issue would have received greater attention. Companies with better gender representation in management might well have caught the problem earlier and could have saved countless lives.

Another of the most notorious examples of institutional or

structural discrimination is the disparity in sentencing guidelines for different forms of cocaine in the United States. Responding to concerns (some have said "hysteria") about a so-called crack epidemic in the 1980s, lawmakers decided the federal penalties for possession of crack cocaine should be one hundred times more severe than the penalties for possession of the same amount of powder cocaine. Thus, someone convicted of holding five grams of crack cocaine would get the same five-year mandatory minimum sentence as someone convicted of possessing five hundred grams of powder cocaine.

The two forms are essentially chemically identical and have virtually the same physiological and addictive properties. But powder cocaine was the stereotypical drug of choice for wealthy white-collar types; crack cocaine was associated with poor and often Black communities.

A 2006 report from the American Civil Liberties Union concluded that "the sentencing disparities in punishing crack cocaine offenses more harshly than powder cocaine offenses unjustly and disproportionately penalize African American defendants for drug trafficking comparable to that of white defendants. Compounding this problem is the fact that whites are disproportionately less likely to be prosecuted for drug offenses in the first place."[26] In 2010, Congress revised the sentencing guidelines down from a one-hundred-to-one disparity to an eighteen-to-one disparity. This was progress, but cocaine sentencing policy remains a form of institutionalized bias and is still an issue today.

The consequences of these forms of institutional bias are huge, yet they don't require psychological bias in the minds of the car executives or the judges who are dealing with these issues. Institutional bias is wired into the way our organizations and institutions work, whether through laws and legislation, rules, policies, or procedures.

Prestigious universities often have what they call "legacy" admissions policies, which give preferential treatment to the children of alumni or donors. Because White people have, on average, had more historical access to higher education and possess more wealth to donate, these systems continue to advantage White students.

In the case of policing, city governments and politicians set policies and priorities that influence where officers are sent on patrol. If these policies send more officers to poor and minority neighborhoods than to predominantly White and wealthy ones, then as a function of numbers alone, there will be more traffic stops—and arrests—of poor and minority people.

These problems can be worsened by technology. If algorithms are trained on data sets of past college admission decisions or prior neighborhood crime rates, they can lead to decisions that will continue to disadvantage members of historically disenfranchised communities.[27] In some cases, these biases are made worse by technology because design features and machine-learning algorithms can obscure sources of bias and give the appearance of objective decision-making.

One place where this occurs is on peer-to-peer platforms. Each year, people around the world book more than seven hundred million Airbnb rentals and take more than ten billion Uber trips. But there is growing evidence of discrimination on these platforms. Airbnb users with Black-sounding names, for example, are less likely to be accepted as guests, and apartments belonging to Black Airbnb hosts are priced 10 percent lower than similar apartments owned by White hosts. It might seem an impossible task to eradicate the biases—implicit or explicit—of the vast number of Airbnb users. But we found that simply changing how the platform presents key information might be enough to reduce discriminatory outcomes.

In a series of experiments led by Katrine Berg Nødtvedt and Hallgeir Sjåstad at the Norwegian School of Economics, we examined solutions for reducing racial bias in the sharing economy.[28] When we gave Norwegian customers the option to rent an Airbnb apartment or hotel, they were 25 percent more likely to choose the apartment when it was hosted by a racial in-group member than when it was hosted by a racial out-group member. However, when we provided a simple cue about trust—a five-star rating from other customers—this pattern of bias completely went away. When these ratings were less visible (or mediocre), people continued to discriminate.

The lesson here is not that we eradicated bias in the minds of potential customers. Instead, we altered the way the platform displayed critical information. The race of the hosts might affect consumers because it is linked to racial stereotypes about whom they should trust. But if crowdsourcing provides alternative, reality-based information about the actual trustworthiness of hosts, guests are happy to stay with people from a different racial background. If companies in the peer-to-peer economy want to reduce racial bias, they should design websites and apps that feature this reputational information more prominently than the identity of the hosts.

Cleaning up our institutions and improving technology to reduce disparate treatment of different groups is a moral imperative. Further, creating fairer and more effective rules, policies, and procedures may have cascading positive consequences beyond the institutions themselves. The existence of transparent, fair, and effective institutions might make people in general less likely to discriminate in favor of their shared groups and social identities.

Earlier, we described the coalitional psychology that our species might have evolved to help us navigate our ancestral environments. People are always on the lookout for allies and wary of potential enemies. Allyship grounded in shared social identities is one way to protect ourselves and to increase the odds that the people we're interacting with are trustworthy and will treat us well. Having loyal friends is one way to hedge our bets in a chaotic world.

But many of the institutions our societies have developed can serve this same function. For example, if you are lucky enough to live in a society with a legal system that works reasonably effectively and fairly, it helps you feel secure in your interactions with a broad array of other people. If you know that, generally speaking, people who rob or defraud others are caught and punished, you can expect that the legal system will act as a deterrent to anyone who might be tempted to rob you. If you know that contracts are enforceable, you can expect to have legal recourse if you are cheated in a transaction.[29]

Without effective institutions, people may opt to restrict their circle of trust to those with whom they already have a connection, either in the form of a personal relationship or through a shared social identity. They may choose to selectively hire, do business, or otherwise affiliate with people like themselves because it feels like a safer bet. But where there are effective institutions that support good behavior across whole societies, the circle of trust can safely open up to include people without prior personal or group connections. Perhaps for this reason, we have found that the more people trust important social institutions, including the government, legal system, and police, the more comfortable they are interacting with members of other racial groups.

We have also found evidence that institution-like structures can reduce implicit biases. In two experiments, we had White students come into the lab and told them that later on in the study, they would play a series of games with other students.[30] They could see from photos that some of the other students were White and some were Black. The games required a level of trust because there was always the possibility that the other students might cheat. But we informed half of the participants that everyone would be monitored by an observer who would punish bad behavior. In other words, someone would play the role of a disinterested enforcer and make it less likely that their partners would cheat.

After we had told them about this setup but before they actually played the games, we had the students complete a measure of implicit racial bias. When White participants expected to play games where someone was monitoring behavior, they showed no implicit preference for White over Black faces. When they expected to play

THE POWER OF US

games without this trust-enhancing feature, however, they showed a typical pattern of pro-White implicit bias.

The results were similar to what we saw when we assigned people to mixed-race teams like the Leopards and the Tigers—implicit racial bias was eliminated. But here, there were no teams. Having an institutional-type structure to promote trust between people reduced bias even in the absence of a shared identity. Promoting trust between people—in this case, in the form of a fairness enforcer—might reduce our need for teams in the first place.

TAKING ACTION

Now, having looked in some depth at the nature of bias—implicit bias especially—it is time to return to the question posed by Senator John Kennedy to Merrick Garland. "Does [implicit bias] mean I'm a racist, no matter what I do or what I think?"

Garland gave a sophisticated response. "That label *racist*," he said, "is not one that I would apply like that. Implicit bias just means that every human being has biases. The point of examining our implicit biases is to bring our conscious mind up to our unconscious mind—and to know when we're behaving in a stereotyped way."

There certainly are beliefs, overtly held, endorsed, even enthusiastically promoted, that are blatantly and obviously racist. Some groups believe it is right to dominate others. The sorts of rapid implicit biases that psychologists have uncovered and that appear to be widespread are not racist in that sense. Indeed, many people are dismayed when they take a bias test and find that their responses indicate a preference for male over female faces, White over Black faces, or younger over older faces, because these biases are at odds with their beliefs about how the world should work. They value egalitarianism and are horrified to learn that a part of their mind seems to harbor very different sentiments.

In our view, the question of whether implicit bias makes you racist (or sexist or ageist or biased against any particular group) is not answered by whether you have bias but by what you do with that information once you know it. If we seek a more just and equitable world, what people are doing to address disparities and discrimination is more important than what score they get on an implicit bias test. In fact, your implicit bias score can change a good deal from one moment to the next (partly as a result of shifting identities and trust cues, as we have discussed), making it an unreliable indicator of your own attitudes anyway. Conversely, it does not matter all that much if politicians do not have a racist bone in their bodies, as they often proclaim, if the decisions they make perpetuate racial disparities.

There is a fear that because implicit bias seems to suggest that people's reactions to different groups are beyond their full conscious control, they are not responsible if they behave in discriminatory ways. This treats implicit bias as an excuse, a "get out of jail free" card.

To counter this, the two of us would go a step further than Merrick Garland did in his congressional testimony. The point of examining bias, implicit and otherwise, is so we can understand that our minds sometimes produce behaviors and outcomes that are inconsistent with our broader beliefs and values. And recognizing this, we can take control, exerting agency to challenge ourselves and others to build a better world.

Of course, changing the deeply rooted inequities embedded in our societies will take significantly more than a simple laboratory manipulation or even a major intervention on the soccer pitch. It will also take more than a quick course of anti-bias training. These can represent important first steps. But, as we discuss in the next chapter, serious and sustained change takes organized and collective action, first to identify and then to root out the structures that produce disparate opportunities and outcomes. It takes solidarity.

CHAPTER 7

FINDING SOLIDARITY

Sylvia Rosalie Jacobson, an associate professor of social work at Florida State University, was making her way home to the United States from Jerusalem in September 1970.[1] Shortly after taking off from Frankfurt, her plane—TWA Flight 741—was hijacked by members of the Popular Front for the Liberation of Palestine (PFLP). Along with one hundred forty-eight other passengers and crew, she was flown to a remote airstrip in the middle of the Jordanian desert.

After a nerve-racking landing, the plane was boarded by members of the PFLP. Illuminated by a flashlight, a female leader delivered a terrifying message: No one would be leaving the desert until the hijackers' demands—including the release of prisoners—had been met. At this moment, Sylvia Jacobson later wrote, "For the first time, we realized that we were all hostages. We had become a community of our own in an unfamiliar environment under threat and stress."[2]

Conditions on the plane slowly deteriorated as the days dragged on. The cooling system broke down. The lavatories were overwhelmed. People fell ill. To make matters much worse, the hijackers began to remove certain passengers. First, non-Jewish women and children were bused to hotels in the capital city of Amman. Then, at irregular intervals, groups of men were taken away to undisclosed destinations, their fates unknown. Eventually, all of the men were removed, leaving many of the remaining women distraught.

Despite the passengers' initial sense of unity in the desert, several sources of division began to emerge. A group of fourteen college students annoyed the other passengers by treating the experience as more of an adventure than an ordeal. Parents with children felt distinct from nonparents without such responsibilities. And then, a stark divide appeared between Jewish parents who allowed their children to eat the nonkosher food provided by their captors and those who did not.

A more menacing division occurred as their captors aggressively differentiated Jewish and American passengers from the rest. This split passengers who held two passports from those with only one. It was to the advantage of dual-passport holders to keep certain social identities concealed. But as repeated searches of the plane turned up these documents and the captors grew more angry, hiding passports seemed to increase everyone's level of danger.

There were fitful attempts at organization and leadership among the passengers that at first went nowhere. Those who tried to take charge of supervising the lavatories or allocating food, for example, were sharply questioned about their legitimacy: "Who gave *you* any special rights?"

Amid the heat and the stress, the confusion and the discord, there were moments of unity when the passengers aboard Flight 741 regained a common sense of shared identity. This occurred when their captors treated them as a whole. When the hijackers and then soldiers trooped through the cabin, the passengers were keenly aware of their common fate. In those moments, Jacobson wrote, "divisiveness was subdued. Despite differences of nationality, religion, race, sorrows, needs, values, resentments, and fears, there was unity in a show of proud indifference, aloofness, and disdain to the inquisitive stares."

Ultimately, the hostages managed to organize themselves when circumstances generated enough of a sense of shared fate and common goals. Toward the end of the fifth day, passengers learned that their water and food was going to be more strictly rationed. They began to coordinate arrangements for using the toilets and allocating the limited water supply. The college students became less insular and started to provide entertainment for the young children. The sense of solidarity tightened.

On September 11, 1970, after five overwhelming days of shifting moods, alliances, and identities, Sylvia Jacobson and most of the other distressed passengers were released to safety. The PFLP blew up the plane the next day. The crisis was not fully resolved until September 30, when the final hostages were freed in exchange for the release of Palestinian and Arab prisoners.

Professor Jacobson, like all the passengers, lived to tell the tale. But being a social scientist by training and a skilled observer of human dynamics, she did not just go on to regale people with her experiences at dinner parties. She published a scientific article about them, drawing insightful lessons about how groups function under conditions of significant duress.

The hijacking illuminates a fascinating set of group dynamics: how situations can activate new identities, how subgroups form and foster conflict, and how shared goals can provide a sense of solidarity and collective purpose, leading people to coordinate and sacrifice in service of the common good.

In this chapter, we will look at what happens when people come together in solidarity. A sense of common identity is key to understanding when people help and support one another. This happens in day-to-day life when people cooperate to achieve common goals, but it can also occur when they forge connections in challenging conditions. Just like the hostage situation described above, there are many instances in which people build new identities in times of stress. The social identities created during events like hijackings and terror attacks—not to mention stressful life situations like serious illnesses (or when a colleague chokes at a cocktail reception)—

can provide a source of cohesion and resilience to tragedy and disaster.

It is often assumed that people look out for themselves in times of danger or threat. Countless Hollywood movies depict panic or rioting in emergency situations. But in reality, this rarely happens. A half-century of research on disasters, protests, and crowd behavior has found that dire circumstances often inspire the formation of shared identities that enable groups to coordinate effective responses to major challenges. Critically, shared identities also allow marginalized and disadvantaged groups, along with their allies, to mobilize against injustice and push for social change.

A CHANCE TO INTERVENE

Like every undergraduate psychology student, Jay had heard the tragic tale of Kitty Genovese, a story first shared breathlessly by the *New York Times*. Jay knew (or thought he knew) that on the night of March 13, 1964,

> for more than half an hour 38 respectable, law-abiding citizens in Queens watched a killer stalk and stab a woman in three separate attacks in Kew Gardens. Twice the sound of their voices and the sudden glow of their bedroom lights interrupted him and frightened him off. Each time he returned, sought her out and stabbed her again. Not one person telephoned the police during the assault; one witness called after the woman was dead.[3]

Exactly where the supposed total of thirty-eight witnesses came from is not clear. But the notion that so many citizens could callously observe the stabbing and murder of a fellow human being without intervening triggered widespread outrage. People decried the decay of civilization and the degradation of life in New York City.[4]

177

As researchers, we have had some of our best ideas pop into our minds as we read the news, and so it was in 1964 for psychologists John Darley and Bibb Latané, who were working in New York City at the time. Based on the tragic story of Kitty Genovese, they developed and tested a hypothesis that they called "the bystander effect."[5] Their hypothesis stated, in essence, that the more bystanders there are in an emergency situation, the less likely any given person is to help.

They theorized that there were at least two reasons why the presence of other people in an emergency can cause an individual not to act. First, it is not always clear what is and is not an emergency, and people often look to others to try to diagnose the situation. When you see that others are not reacting, you might assume that it is because they know it is not an emergency. This is a big problem if they happen to have reached precisely the same conclusion by gauging *your* reaction, or lack of it. This is known as *pluralistic ignorance*—when no one knows what is going on but assumes that everyone else does.

Second, if people somehow overcome this mutual state of ignorance to recognize an emergency situation for what it is, they may still fail to act due to a *diffusion of responsibility*, in which everyone assumes that someone else should take or perhaps already has taken care of it.

Darley and Latané designed clever laboratory experiments to test their idea. In one experiment, someone faked a seizure. In another, smoke began billowing under a door. They observed how participants responded to these crises when they were alone versus in the presence of other people who did nothing. Sure enough, people were less likely to help when there were others around than when they were alone.

Jay learned about pluralistic ignorance and diffusion of responsibility as an undergraduate student at the University of Alberta. Around the same time, a group of young people, unimpeded by others, attacked an innocent man on the Edmonton subway, once again prompting cries from the public about decaying civilization and big city depravity. In response, Jay wrote a letter to the local newspaper pointing out that the failure of other people to stop the attack may have stemmed, in part, from the bystander effect. He also argued that knowing more about human psychology in these situations might help people overcome these sorts of barriers and take action.

Little did he know that before long, he would have a chance to put this theory to the test.

Jay moved from Alberta to the University of Toronto to complete his PhD in social psychology. One day, he got off the subway after an afternoon of Christmas shopping and was about to leave the station when he noticed a young man running in the opposite direction. The man, who appeared to be about twenty years old, hurdled over the turnstiles without buying a ticket and jumped down a stairwell.

A few seconds later, the young man returned, dragging a woman much smaller than himself up the stairs. He slammed her against the wall and yelled in her face. She was crying as he grabbed her shoulders and shook her violently. Dozens of commuters noticed the commotion and craned their necks to see what was going on. But when they saw what was happening, most averted their eyes and walked past in a rush to catch their evening trains.

Jay ran to report what was happening to a Toronto City Transit employee behind a wall of plexiglass. As the transit official called security, Jay wondered if he had done enough. He sized up the man, who seemed bigger than him and was clearly in a rage. But knowing about the bystander effect, Jay had a sense that pluralistic ignorance and diffusion of responsibility might be stopping others from intervening. His heart was racing, his physiological fight-or-flight response fully engaged, and in that moment he decided to swallow his fear and intervene.

As Jay walked over to the couple, another man joined him, a similarly anxious-looking stranger. They briefly made eye contact and exchanged a nod of understanding before confronting the violent man and telling him to leave the woman alone.

THE POWER OF US

The furious attacker turned around and yelled, "Mind your own business!" He reached into his pocket, and Jay's heart dropped. Was he reaching for a knife? Something worse? Fortunately, it was just a quarter. The man threw the coin and said, "Call someone who cares!"

When the man realized that the two bystanders were not going to leave, he uttered a few threats and stormed off. Jay and his fellow helper escorted the young woman down the stairs to the subway platform and asked if she wanted them to wait with her until security arrived. She declined, saying she simply wanted to go home. She felt safe on her own now that the violent man had left.

Moments later, they heard the train coming. Jay and his compatriot left the woman and walked back toward the stairs to make sure that the attacker could not sneak onto the train and follow her home. Just as they feared, as the subway train pulled into the station and hundreds of commuters surged toward the tracks, the man jumped down the stairwell once again and raced toward the woman.

He screamed at her not to get on the train, but she stepped on. Just as the doors were about to close, the man tried to jump on too. Without thinking, Jay and his compatriot grabbed the man and wrestled him to the ground. As they struggled to hold him without getting punched or spit on, they realized that the conductor, seeing the commotion, had stopped the train. They looked up and saw hundreds of commuters staring at them. The train was frozen and the platform was completely empty, but no one stepped off to help.

Jay again thought to himself, *This is the bystander effect!* And he realized that he needed to explain the situation to the crowd and ask them to help. He needed to break through the pluralistic ignorance and diffusion of responsibility that were holding these people in place. He did so, which led two other strangers to get off the train to help. Together they held the abusive man down until two burly security guards arrived and took over.

Knowing about the bystander effect might help people overcome the psychological barriers to helping in emergencies, as it did for

Jay. But we now also know that neither the tale of Kitty Genovese nor the bystander effect is as straightforward as was long believed.[6] Some of the neighbors who heard Kitty Genovese's cries for help the night of her death did intervene in one way or another. Although they were not sure what was happening, several shouted out of their windows and temporarily scared off the attacker. Some neighbors, including a boy who would later become a New York City police officer, reported calling the police during the attack. That the police never responded might have had something to do with the fact that there was no centralized 911 system in the United States until 1968, four years later. Before that, each police station, firehouse, and hospital had its own number, and there was no standardized system for receiving or responding to calls from the public.

The bystander effect might give the inaccurate impression that helping is very rare in emergency situations. Research suggests, however, that people actually do intervene in many, perhaps most, emergencies. A recent study, for example, examined surveillance-camera footage of aggressive incidents in urban areas in the Netherlands, South Africa, and Britain.[7] The researchers found that out of 219 public conflicts between two or more people, at least one observer intervened in 199 of them—that is, 91 percent of the time.

As you might expect, the more people who are around, the greater likelihood there is that *someone* will step forward, just by virtue of sheer numbers. But this doesn't mean the chance of *you* intervening increases. It is important to understand this difference: the more people who are around, the better the chance that someone in a crowd will eventually notice something amiss and take action. But the probability of any given person in that situation doing something may still be quite low unless something triggers that person to help.

Understanding pluralistic ignorance and the diffusion of responsibility are still useful for understanding when people are and are not likely to help. If people do not intervene because they are not sure whether what they are seeing is an emergency, it leads to the somewhat counterintuitive prediction that they should be less susceptible to the bystander effect in more dangerous situations. When things are really dangerous, it should be more clearly obvious that an emergency is real and perhaps that multiple people are needed to help. Consistent with this, a meta-analysis of over one hundred bystander studies found that in more dangerous emergencies, the presence of other people did less to deter people from helping.[8]

In Jay's case, his understanding of the bystander effect—and perhaps his burgeoning identity as a social psychologist—caused him to intervene while others did not. But obviously, you don't have to be a social psychologist to intervene! Other identities matter too when it comes to helping. Indeed, simply recognizing that you share a social identity with someone seems to be a significant cause of helping.

EXPANDING OUR MORAL CIRCLES

How much we offer help to other people, like so much else, depends on whether we see them as sharing a part of our identities. The philosopher Peter Singer refers to this idea as a "moral circle," the boundaries of which determine who is deserving of our concern—and, of course, who is not.[9] Many things that are now considered fundamental human rights—free speech, freedom from oppression, voting—have expanded over time from privileges possessed only by a few elites in the ruling classes to larger groups. The expansion of rights to women, ethnic, racial, and religious minorities, the LGBTQ community, and so on can be understood as a widening of the moral circle.

The boundaries of our identities are not fixed; they can vary across time and situations based on what is most salient. While Martin Luther King Jr. might have been right when he said, "The arc of the moral universe is long, but it bends toward justice," the people we feel a responsibility to help and care for in any given moment is fluid.

British football (or, to Americans, soccer) fans do not have the best reputation, but they are willing to help their own. Mark Levine and colleagues invited Manchester United fans to his psychological laboratory at the University of Lancaster.[10] They arrived and completed a series of tasks designed to remind them of how much they loved Manchester United and being a fan of the team. Then they were asked to walk to another building to complete the study.

On the way they encountered an emergency. A young man ran out across the path ahead of them, tripped, fell, and clutched his ankle, moaning in pain. Would they help this man in distress?

The clumsy stranger—secretly in cahoots with the experimenters—was always the same person. But his identity was not always the same. One group of fans encountered a young man in a plain, unadorned shirt. Another group saw him wearing a Manchester United jersey, exhibiting his allegiance to the Red Devils. And a third group met a fan of Liverpool, which, in the eyes of many Manchester United fans, is their greatest rival.

This simple difference in jerseys was pivotal. Whereas 92 percent of Manchester United fans helped the injured stranger when he was wearing a Manchester United jersey, only 30 percent stopped to help if he was a Liverpool fan. Importantly, this lack of helping seemed to be less about an aversion to assisting the fan of a rival club than about the absence of a shared identity, because only 33 percent helped the stranger wearing a plain shirt!

Okay, fine, you're thinking. *Manchester United fans are parochial wankers unwilling to lend a hand to anyone outside their own group.* But not so fast...

In a second study, Levine and colleagues repeated the experiment but changed what the Manchester United fans were asked to think about when they arrived in the lab. This time, they completed tasks designed to remind them of how much they loved "the beautiful game" and being a *football fan in general,* activating a larger and more inclusive identity than their specific club.

Everything else in the study proceeded as before, but the results changed rather dramatically. Now the Manchester United fans were just as willing to help an injured Liverpool fan as they were a Manchester United fan. However, they were still unlikely to help the hapless stranger without a logo on his shirt. In other words, the active social identities of these fans were bigger than before. Their moral circle was larger, and thus they were helpful to a broader swath of humanity, albeit only those who loved football.

In some ways, this mirrors the experience of the hijacked passengers in the Jordanian desert. When they felt a shared sense of identity, they readily cooperated. But when they were divided over food, parenting, or passports, they were less willing to help one another. The same people who act uncaringly in one situation might be generous and supportive in another, and shifts in identity can help explain why.

First-aid training programs often focus on how to recognize emergencies and how to respond. But helping is not just about knowing what to do. As this research shows, it starts with whom we identify with enough to want to help, especially in dangerous or frightening situations.

GROUPS IN POTENTIA

As we have seen, different situations can activate one or another of the different identities we hold, with significant consequences for how we think, feel, and act. When you're at a football match, crowded into a stadium with fellow fans, your team identity, rather than your occupational, family, or religious identity, is likely at the forefront of your mind. You hold a set of existing identities, and circumstances bring them in and out of focus. Sometimes, however, the situations we find ourselves in may bring entirely new identities into being.

As we talked about in chapter 1, there's an important distinction to be made between *collections* of people—sets of individuals who happen to be in the same place at the same time—and *psychological groups* of people. The former merely coexist in a common space; the latter share a sense of identity. They know that together they are a meaningful entity, something larger than the individuals the set is composed of.

Collections of people are groups in potentia, lying latent, pending events. Whether passengers on a plane, diners in a restaurant, or neighbors in a suburb, collections of people can become groups when events conspire to create shared social identities. These circumstances might be planned and deliberate, as when someone forms a neighborhood group to unite and organize the local community. Or they might be completely unplanned and even undesired, as when a plane is hijacked or a disaster strikes.

Such a disaster occurred during the morning commute in London on July 7, 2005, when terrorists attacked the city's vast transportation network. Suicide bombers detonated three bombs on underground trains and a fourth on a double-decker bus. Fifty-two people, including the terrorists, were killed and more than seven hundred were injured.

After the bombs exploded, thousands of passengers, many of whom were wounded, were left stunned, surrounded by smoke, darkness, and debris. In this horrific situation, one might have expected mass panic—people pushing and shoving each other out of the way, abandoning the casualties in a mad rush to escape. Pandemonium. Chaos.

But that's not what happened. British psychologist John Drury, who has conducted intensive investigations into how crowds of people respond during emergencies, including the London bombings, believes that there are four key lessons to be learned about what happens during disasters.[11]

First, panic and overreaction are rare. Sylvia Jacobson similarly noted an absence of panic in her account of the hijacking. Passengers

185

exhibited shock, fear, depression, and stunned disbelief at what was happening, but at no point did they lose their heads. Second, it is common for survivors to help and support one another. Third, a great deal of this help and support comes about because survivors possess, in that moment, a shared sense of identity. And fourth, the way that emergency responders and authorities treat a crowd shapes how the crowd reacts, in large part by affecting that shared sense of identity.

After the London bombings, Drury and his colleagues interviewed survivors and scoured public accounts in which people talked about what had happened.[12] Although it was not uncommon for people to use the word *panic,* the term was used most often to describe a natural emotional state of fear and shock rather than disordered or frantic behavior. People's demeanor was frequently characterized as calm, orderly, and controlled despite the turmoil around them. One interviewee said:

> It was quite a calm calm evenly dispersed evacuation there wasn't people running down the train screaming their heads [off]. It was very calm and obviously there was people crying but generally most sort of people were calm in that situation, which I found amazing.

In addition, interviewees reported a sense of unity with others:

> I felt that we're all in the same boat together...it was a stressful situation and we're all in it together and the best way to get out of it was to help each other...yeah so I felt exactly I felt quite close to the people near me.

Consistent with the research on shared identity and helping, mutual support was common. Newspapers carried stories about fifty-seven people who described helping others and seventeen people who described being helped; one hundred forty additional people witnessed acts of helping. Only three reports included eyewitnesses describing selfish behavior.

Emergencies and disasters are extreme events, but we can learn much from them about how identity dynamics operate under more normal, less terrifying circumstances. A sense of common fate produces a shared identity, the knowledge that we, together, are part of a group. That shared identity produces solidarity and the ability to work together collectively. When they cohere, shared identities become foundations on which people can coordinate and cooperate.

ON THE SAME WAVELENGTH

We have argued throughout this book that one of the fundamental benefits of shared identities is that they enable groups of people to achieve things that they could not on their own. In some instances, it is obvious that working together allows us to accomplish remarkable things. Unless people can coordinate, they are not going to build a cathedral, play a symphony, or vaccinate an entire population. But in other cases, it is not so obvious that working together is for the best. Surely, certain kinds of tasks are better done on one's own or at least motivated by one's own individual interests.

In recent research, we have started to put this question to the test and investigate what happens to our brains when we work together in solidarity, as opposed to as individuals. We wanted to examine if *psychological groups* of people would find it easier to get on the same neural wavelength and by doing so outperform mere *collections* of people—sets of individuals who happen to be in the same place at the same time.

In one study led by PhD student Diego Reinero, we invited 174 people to the lab to complete a series of quite difficult tasks.[13] In one task, for example, they were given a list of supplies and asked to rank them in order of importance for surviving a plane crash in the heart

187

of winter. Some of the choices are counterintuitive unless you are a survival expert, and it takes careful reasoning to make good decisions.

For every session, four participants came to the lab at the same time. Before we let them loose with the problem-solving tasks, we randomly assigned each set of four to either complete the tasks collaboratively as a group or try their best as individuals.

To create feelings of solidarity in the collaborative groups, we told them that they would be competing against other teams on the problem-solving tasks. We also put some money on the line: if their team was ranked in the top 5 percent of all teams, they would receive a two-hundred-dollar bonus to be split equally among them (fifty dollars each). We then asked them to create a team name and had them tap along in unison to some funky music while facing one another. Moving to music is an ancient tool for helping people feel a sense of collective purpose.

In contrast, participants assigned to work as individuals were told they would be working alone and competing against other individuals on the tasks. Individuals ranked in the top 5 percent would receive a fifty-dollar bonus. We then asked each of them to create a personal code name and had them turn away from the group to tap along to the same music as they privately listened to it on their own headphones. This was designed to make them feel that they were in a dog-eat-dog world of individual competition.

You might notice some uncomfortable parallels between this condition and organizations or workplaces you are familiar with. Many companies, schools, and even families structure their incentives a lot like our individualistic condition. People compete against one another for awards and cultivate individual identities. In open-plan office spaces, many employees don headphones to tune out others and curate their own mental experiences.

It is often assumed that people perform best when they can maximize their own outcomes. But knowing what we do about identity, we suspected that people might actually perform better when they were working together in solidarity than alone in competition with one another.

As participants prepared for their tasks, our research team placed a small headset on each of them to record the electrical activity of their brains as they completed the study. These devices are fairly small and fit on the head like a small crown. Once the study was under way, many participants seemed to completely forget about them.

As they worked through the tasks, we were able to measure participants' patterns of brain activity to see if they were, quite literally, on the same wavelength as other members of their group. We compared each person's brain activity throughout the study to the patterns exhibited by everyone else completing the tasks at the same time in order to assess levels of neural synchrony. To what extent were their brains firing in similar ways at the same time?

The first thing we noticed when we analyzed the data was that the groups working together as teams outperformed the sets of individuals on almost every task. They came to better solutions on the survival task, as well as on sudoku puzzles, photographic memory, brainstorming, and word unscrambling, than the average individual working alone. Being on a team consistently produced better results than working alone.

People also cooperated more when they were in a meaningful group than when they were merely part of a set of individuals. We told everyone in each session that ten dollars of their winnings could be donated to the collective. All of the money would be pooled together, doubled, and then split equally among all four people. So if all four donated their full ten dollars, each person would walk away with twenty dollars. We found that 74 percent of people in the team condition donated the full ten dollars to their group, but only 51 percent of people in the individual condition did the same.

In other words, teams outperformed individuals on almost every element of collective decision-making. The only task where teams performed worse than individuals was a simple typing assignment in which working together and coordinating responses slowed them down. Teamwork was not always the solution, but it certainly worked better most of the time.

When we looked at brain activity, we noticed a similar pattern. At first, people who were working together in groups were no more synchronized than those who were working as individuals. But as the study went on, the brains of people working together started to mirror one another. By the end of the study, there was a clear difference in the degree of brain synchrony for teams versus individuals.

Even more important, this brain synchrony was related to performance! Teams that were more synchronized had the best performance on the tasks—they were better at collective decision-making. While they were almost certainly not aware of it, being on the same neural wavelength was related to their success.

Similar dynamics are at play in the classroom, yet another place where people can see themselves as a collection of individuals or as part of a group. Led by our collaborator Suzanne Dikker, we worked with a high-school biology class to measure their brain activity over an entire semester.[14] Every week for roughly three months, Suzanne went to the class and placed headsets on a group of twelve students. We recorded their brain activity as they learned about neuroscience.

One of the biggest challenges for a teacher is keeping a roomful of kids engaged as they make their way through complex material. In our study, the teacher took a variety of approaches, including reading aloud, showing videos, lecturing, and leading discussions, to help the students learn. And while the students learned, we examined when they were on the same wavelength.

As it turns out, viewing videos and taking part in discussions were not only the most enjoyable elements of the class, they were also the moments when students had the most similar patterns of brain activity. As synchrony increased for the entire group, they were more engaged and rated the class more positively. Interestingly, we also found that when a student made brief social contact with another student before the lesson, their two brains were more likely to be in sync during the class and they felt closer to each other that day. Those fleeting moments of connection seemed to put people on the same wavelength.

Across these studies, getting people on the same wavelength was key to group decision-making, learning, and cooperation. They speak to the sort of everyday situations where greater awareness of the consequences of shared identities and social connections can be truly beneficial.

But shared identities have broader societal-level contributions to make as well, particularly when it comes to social change and the pursuit of greater justice in the world. Martin Luther King Jr.'s long arc bending toward justice has been the inexorable result not of human enlightenment, but of a series of difficult battles—often led by those without access to equal justice—for the expansion of human rights and other collective goods. Change happens when people find solidarity with one another and fight for it.

FIGHTING FOR CHANGE

Shared identities help marginalized groups and their allies organize and mobilize for change. As we have seen, it is possible for people to form social identities around just about anything. For long periods of history, however, large collections of people suffering under oppression—serfs, slaves, members of stigmatized groups and castes—have not had much chance to mobilize around common interests. This raises crucial questions: When do people who belong to marginalized and disenfranchised social categories rally around these as social identities and push for change? And what makes their collective action successful?

Human beings' most important social identities are created around and fostered by shared traditions, rituals, histories, myths

191

THE POWER OF US

and stories, memories of accomplishments, and joys. But they are also forged by adversity, hardship, and the ways people are treated and mistreated by others. When people come to realize that their opportunities and outcomes in life are limited because they happen to belong to a particular group and that those limitations are illegitimate, it tends to generate a sense of common fate and shared identity.

This phenomenon is powerfully illustrated by a demonstration conducted by author and educator Jackson Katz.[15] He first asks the men in the room: "What steps do you guys take, on a daily basis, to prevent yourselves from being sexually assaulted?" This often leads to an awkward pause. Most often, the men have nothing to say. Then he asks the women the same thing. Hands immediately shoot up, and women share the many and routine safety precautions they take every day, like holding their keys so they can be used for self-defense, checking the back seats of cars before getting in, always carrying a cell phone, avoiding going out alone at night, carrying pepper spray, parking in well-lit areas, and on and on.

This exercise reveals the very serious risks that women face (and that many men are oblivious to), but it also indicates something about how many women experience their gender identity. Most men probably do not think much about their gender on a day-to-day basis simply because being male does not put them at risk. But the enormous list of precautions routinely taken by women indicates that many women possess a more chronic awareness of their gender because of the danger posed to them by, for the most part, men.

Social identities are strengthened and are more likely to become a rallying point for change when members of disadvantaged or oppressed groups perceive the social system they are in to be *impermeable* and *illegitimate*.[16] When people believe that a system is *impermeable,* they perceive that their place and experience in society is bound to their group and that they are not free to thrive as fully as the members of other, more advantaged groups. When they believe the system to be *illegitimate,* they regard this state of affairs as fundamentally unjust. In the case of gender violence, women encounter significantly more danger than men do—an experience that is bound to their group membership. Through movements like #MeToo, the reality of this discrepancy in the experiences of men and women is increasingly recognized and regarded as horrific and utterly unjustifiable.

The infamous "glass ceiling" that prevents women from rising to executive ranks in corporate life is another example of an illegitimate impermeability. However, as the term *glass ceiling* implies, group-based barriers are not always obviously apparent, and there are often forces working to keep them invisible. One such force is a strong tendency in many societies to attribute outcomes solely to individual agency. There is also an inclination to see the world and the things that happen in it as essentially fair and to rationalize the systems in which we live—a process known as system justification.[17]

It's as if many people have an implicit belief in karma. When bad things happen to people, others often assume that they must have deserved it in some way. This can produce victim-blaming, when people are held responsible and even shamed or punished for circumstances and outcomes beyond their control.[18] This is common in sexual-assault cases when the public—and sometimes even the legal system—places as much or more blame on women who have been victimized than on perpetrators. More generally, the propensity to individualize outcomes can cause people to hear about group-based disparities in wages or health or justice and write them off as individual choices or failures.

She got harassed at a bar? *Well, she shouldn't wear clothes like that. And why was she out so late anyway?*

She earns less than him? *Well, she didn't negotiate hard enough.*

He got pulled over and searched by the cops again? *Well, if he didn't drive that flashy car, he wouldn't draw attention.*

When people make these sorts of individual rather than situational attributions, it distracts from systemic or structural factors that negatively affect the members of some groups more than others.

Another force pushing against recognition of illegitimate treatment based on the social categories people belong to is a phenomenon known as tokenism.[19] Except in the most brutally repressive regimes, at least a few members of disadvantaged groups often manage to overcome some of the barriers in front of them and succeed. Tokenism occurs when these individuals are held up as evidence that the system is fair and permeable after all. Any problems that society might have had are thus considered things of the past. Look, we have a female CEO. Or a gay mayor. Or a Black president.

When Barack Obama was elected president in 2008, at least some people saw it as a sign that the United States had moved beyond problems of race. A study by Cheryl Kaiser, a professor at the University of Washington, and colleagues found people reported that contemporary racism was less of a problem in the United States after Obama's election.[20] They were also less supportive than they had been before the election of policies that reduced racial inequality. In their minds, President Obama's success seemed to prove that the system was just and fair.

In these and other ways, people engage in system justification, rationalizing inequalities to themselves and to others. In our own research on the topic, we have found that this system-justifying tendency can lead people to judge racial minorities more harshly and resist equal rights for the LGBTQ community.[21] When people identify with an oppressive system, they are often motivated to maintain it.

To push past these sorts of system-justifying forces, disenfranchised group members and their allies engage in an often slow and grinding process of consciousness-raising. *Yes, this is a real problem. It is really wrong. It is systemic. This is not a one-off incident. And together we can do something about it.*

The #MeToo and #BlackLivesMatter movements are recent

examples of successful—but still ongoing—consciousness-raising. Both have involved significant organization and on-the-streets protest, as well as organic online activism. Some people criticize online components of movements as mere hashtag protest or "slacktivism," but social media paired with cell phone videos has been a game-changer for these civil rights issues.

Videos, especially of police brutality against Black and other minority citizens, have opened the eyes of people around the world to the astonishing frequency of these events. Between 2014, when New York City police officers killed Eric Garner, and 2020, the percentage of Americans who believe that the police are more likely to use excessive force against Black people than others rose from 33 percent to 57 percent.[22] Similarly, the MeToo hashtag has allowed women to document and demonstrate the prevalence of sexual harassment and assault in societies worldwide.

Importantly, the consciousness-raising accomplished by movements like BLM and MeToo doesn't affect only the identities and allegiances of disadvantaged or disenfranchised group members. Men can also be shocked and appalled by what they learn about the sexual harassment and inequitable treatment experienced by women. So too can White people come to understand that the social system is structured in such a way that it tends to benefit them (or give them the benefit of the doubt) more than it does Black people and members of other racial minority groups. They too can come to perceive these disparities as fundamentally illegitimate and advocate for social change.

Of course, not every male, White, or otherwise advantaged person comes to see it this way, and mere knowledge of disparities is not enough to create cross-group allyship. But when these shifts in perception cause shifts in identification, we end up with movements for change that look like the BLM marches of 2020, when people of many different races, ages, genders, religions, and cultural backgrounds raised their voices in a moment of solidarity.[23]

TAKING TO THE STREETS

As we were writing this book in 2020, protests in support of the Black Lives Matter movement spread across the United States and around the world. The protests began in Minneapolis as people demanded the arrest of the police officers involved in the killing of George Floyd. Sparked by anguish and anger at the unjust death of yet another Black citizen and rallying against police violence more generally, the BLM protests grew over the summer into what crowd-counters believe were the largest protests in American history. People also marched in cities as far apart as London, Toronto, Amsterdam, Sydney, and Rio de Janeiro.

The vast majority of these protests were peaceful, but some were not, and there were instances of looting as well as violent confrontations between protesters and the police. As support for the protests grew, so did backlash, and it was clear that what people saw in these events was perceived through the lenses of their own identities. Where some saw peaceful crowds exercising their rights, others saw unruly mobs. Where some saw overly aggressive cops, others saw officers doing their duty. Once again, identities shaped perceptions and created their own distinct realities.

But it is not all perception. What actually happens during protests and the chances that they remain peaceful or become violent has a great deal to do with identity dynamics. In particular, the responses of protesters are often affected by the way they are treated by authorities. Relations between these groups shape their senses of identity as well as norms about appropriate courses of action. In this regard, events during the 2020 BLM protests mirrored patterns observed during many prior protests.[24]

In 2011, for example, British police shot and killed Mark Duggan, a multiracial man, in Tottenham, a suburb of London. Following his death, riots broke out in Tottenham and then spread to other suburbs and cities around England. There was looting and arson, and five people were killed. Thousands of people were arrested in angry confrontations with police.

Although unrest spread across neighborhoods and among cities, it did not spread everywhere. Why not? A report on what became known as the London Riots found that the areas where riots occurred had higher levels of deprivation, as indicated by factors like lower incomes, poorer health, and more barriers to education. Deprived areas also tended to have longer riots and more arrests.[25] Areas with riots had also experienced higher rates of police stops and searches of their residents during the preceding two and a half years.

Deprivation and frequent negative encounters with the police were an important part of the context in many locations when Mark Duggan was killed. These were places where people already distrusted the police and saw themselves in opposition to the authorities. When Duggan was shot, these conditions provided the foundation for a social identity to emerge in which communities perceived themselves as allied against the police. Unrest spread as people across London and other cities around the UK came to see themselves as sharing a common fate, bound together by their treatment at the hands of the authorities.

The actions of the police further fostered and shaped this identity. The first riot in Tottenham did not occur until two days after Duggan's death. On that Saturday, Duggan's family and friends led a protest outside the Tottenham police station. The protest was peaceful until the police were perceived to assault a young woman in the crowd. It was at this critical point that "violence against the police first became normative" and spread.

Most protests, of course, are not about the police, or at least they do not start off that way. People rally to oppose an oil pipeline or a garbage dump. They take to the streets against an unpopular tax or a political scandal. The police are called in to maintain order and project state authority. Most people who attend protests or engage in other forms of collective action are there to pursue a change-oriented goal that they believe is important. They are not there to loot, riot, or take part in violent confrontations with the police.

Sometimes, of course, there are a few individuals who are looking for trouble, and media coverage often focuses on people smashing windows or looting shops because it is newsworthy. But the evidence suggests that protesters left to their own devices often stop these people or push them out. Crowds coordinate around norms for appropriate behavior and enforce them. They can and do actively police themselves. But this dynamic breaks down swiftly in the face of aggressive actions from the police.[26]

During the BLM protests of 2020, we saw police around the world do the right things; we also saw police do the wrong things, at least if promoting peaceful protest was the goal. We saw officers in ordinary uniforms marching alongside protesters, taking a knee, comforting people in tears, and stopping to help people who had been injured. In these situations, conflict de-escalated. We saw police chiefs provide platforms for community leaders who, while tremendously upset, sought to channel their communities' anger toward nonviolent action. All of these serve to break down the "us" versus "them" distinction and provide agency within crowds to manage themselves.

But we also saw police officers approach peaceful crowds wearing riot gear and driving military-style vehicles. We saw officers charge at civilians, seemingly without provocation. We saw police shoot tear gas and rubber bullets at protesters and members of the media who had broken no rules and posed no threat. These actions harden the "us" versus "them" distinction and can shift norms within groups of protesters from peaceful to violent action. And when videos of these actions go viral, it can be like throwing a match on gasoline.

By aggressively treating crowds as if they are dangerous monoliths, the police induce an experience of common fate that can create identities bound together in opposition to the authorities. The preemptive use of violence by the police is often seen as illegitimate and may justify, in the eyes of many, the use of violence by protesters in return. The troublemakers that had been pushed out may start to gain credibility and influence within the crowd. More peacefully oriented protesters may now be pushed out or may choose to adopt the new, more violent norms.

Overly aggressive police responses, in other words, often escalate violence unnecessarily, turning crowds into mobs and protests into riots. Perhaps police hope that the intimidating use of force will serve as a deterrent, causing protesters to scatter and not return. But this neglects the power of social identities. When the actions of authorities are widely regarded as illegitimate, it unifies people in opposition against them.

WHOSE SIDE ARE WE ON?

Ultimately, perceptions of whose actions and whose claims hold the greatest legitimacy influence the success or failure of movements for social change. Social movements succeed at instigating change when sufficient numbers of people with the power to make it happen come on board. In different contexts, these might be members of the voting public, members of the media, politicians, or even security and police forces themselves. By default, these third parties tend to support the status quo or at least are not often motivated to oppose it. Change happens more quickly when their loyalties shift.

The tactics used by protesters and resistance movements seem to matter a great deal for instigating change. Political scientists Erica Chenoweth and Maria Stephan examined the effectiveness of social movements in countries around the world between the years 1900 and 2006.[27] They compared the success rate of violent versus nonviolent campaigns. Contrary to the intuition that deep changes come about only at the barrel of a gun, they found that over this long period of history, nonviolent campaigns were significantly more successful than violent ones. Whereas violent campaigns succeeded 26 percent of the time, nonviolent ones succeeded about 53 percent of the time! Nonviolence was twice as effective at producing change.

Nonviolence worked for at least two reasons. First, it made movements more attractive to potential supporters, helping them build more inclusive social identities. Nonviolent tactics are perceived as more legitimate, bringing more people into the movement and gaining more support from outsiders. Second, when authorities used violence against nonviolent movements, it tended to backfire, increasing sympathy and support for protesters and activists. This reduced the number of people who identified with the police and increased the number who identified with the protesters.

Allegiances begin to shift. And in places where movements aspire to change regimes—to replace leaders and topple dictators—the allegiances of the security forces themselves are often pivotal. Police officers and members of the military are more likely to shift their loyalties when they are unwilling to take more violent action against peaceful civilians and fellow citizens. Regimes fall when they refuse to do so.

It is critical to note that nonviolent resistance is not passive resistance. Groups pushing for change need to draw attention to their cause. They need headlines. They need to raise consciousness. Often this means civil disobedience, causing a ruckus, breaking the law. We may see people doing things that ordinarily we do not like: spraying graffiti, blocking roads and railway lines, occupying parks and office buildings. These actions are designed not only to challenge people in power, but to get public attention and ultimately change public opinion.

This leads to what Matthew Feinberg and colleagues refer to as "the activist's dilemma."[28] Protest actions like blocking highways and vandalizing properties can be effective at applying pressure to institutions and raising awareness, but these same actions may also undermine popular support for social movements. Finding the right balance is critical for instigating effective social change.

The media is also often crucial. Most people do not observe protests or other forms of collective action directly; they hear about them through news outlets. The way that the media frames protest and resistance—whom they define as the "good guys" and the "bad guys"—plays a key role in shaping public opinion. And the media too is responsive to protest tactics.

A recent analysis by Omar Wasow, professor of politics, looked at different types of protests during the U.S. civil rights movement and the kinds of headlines that appeared in major newspapers.[29] He found that nonviolent protests were associated with more headlines about civil rights and with greater agreement that civil rights was an important issue in subsequent public opinion polls. Violent protests, in contrast, were associated with more headlines about riots and stronger public endorsement of social control.

His analysis suggests that nonviolent protests in a U.S. county increased the number of people voting for Democrats (who were generally in favor of expanding civil rights) by about 1.6 percent. But violent protests decreased the number of people voting for Democrats by anywhere from 2.2 to 5.4 percent.

Most of the time and for the majority of social injustices, most people are among those third parties whose allegiances can tip the scale one way or the other. Even if they are the activists in one battle for change, they are the observers in many others. And as an observer, each person must ask him- or herself these fundamental questions: *With whom do I stand? Whose cause has greater legitimacy? Who is on the side of justice and the moral arc of history? With whom do I identify?*

CHAPTER 8

FOSTERING DISSENT

Helicopter gunner Ron Ridenhour began to hear the "dark and bloody" rumors in late April 1968. Hanging around U.S. headquarters in Vietnam, Ridenhour ran into a buddy he had met during aviation training. His friend had a disturbing story to tell. About a month earlier, troops belonging to Charlie Company had conducted what should have been an ordinary strike on a suspected Vietcong stronghold. But when they choppered into the village of My Lai, something went terribly awry.[1]

To their surprise, the soldiers found only a tiny settlement—trees, huts, and farm animals—occupied not by enemy combatants but by women, children, and men too old to fight. In the hours that followed, American troops slaughtered the defenseless villagers. Large numbers of Vietnamese civilians were mercilessly killed, mown down by machine guns, executed with pistols, or blown up by grenades thrown into their homes. Some estimates said that more than five hundred people died in My Lai. The hamlet was burned to the ground.

Shocked, Ridenhour had trouble believing what he had heard. But over the course of the next year, he pieced together bits of the story from soldiers who had been part of Charlie Company themselves or who knew men who were. The details he heard were horrible and horribly consistent. He assembled the facts as best he could, and upon his return to the United States at the end of his tour of duty, Ridenhour wrote it all down in a letter. He sent his letter to thirty people, including members of Congress, the president, and officials at the Pentagon:

> Exactly what did, in fact, occur in the village of [My Lai] in March 1968 I do not know for certain, but I am convinced it was very black indeed. I remain irrevocably persuaded that if you and I do truly believe in the principles of justice and the equality of every man, however humble, before the law, that form the very backbone that this country is founded on, then we must press forward a widespread and public investigation of this matter with all our combined efforts.[2]

Ridenhour's letter triggered an internal investigation by the army that resulted in several indictments. Ultimately only one man, Lieutenant William Calley, was convicted of crimes committed in My Lai. When the American public became aware of the massacre and the evidence that it had been covered up, the stories divided the country. Public support for the war in Vietnam was further eroded. But at the same time, many people reacted angrily to Ron Ridenhour and to other whistleblowers for taking actions they saw as unpatriotic treachery that undermined the troops. In 1974, six years after the slaughter in My Lai, William Calley, the only person ever held accountable, was pardoned by President Richard Nixon.

Ron Ridenhour went on to become an esteemed investigative journalist. Later reflecting on his experience uncovering the atrocities committed by soldiers at My Lai, he wrote, "The question most often put to me was not why they had done it, but why I had done it."[3]

In this chapter, we explain how social identities motivate people to express dissent. Although most people assume that good group members comply with social norms and suppress criticism of their groups, our research suggests that the deepest form of group loyalty often involves the expression of disagreement when people think it is necessary to salvage the values and goals of their in-group.

A RIGHT AND A DUTY

Among nations, America is a country that knows the value of civil disobedience, which makes the negative reactions elicited by dissenters and whistleblowers like Ron Ridenhour all the more surprising. From the Boston Tea Party to the civil rights movement, protest is part of the American DNA. The publication of the Declaration of Independence in 1776 founded the United States in a blazing act of dissent, upholding rebellion as not just a right but a duty:

> We hold these truths to be self-evident, that all men are created equal, that they are endowed by their Creator with certain unalienable Rights, that among these are Life, Liberty and the pursuit of Happiness...But when a long train of abuses and usurpations...evinces a design to reduce them under absolute Despotism, it is their right, it is their duty, to throw off such Government, and to provide new Guards for their future security.

The Congress of the original thirteen colonies may have had King George III in mind, but their words went on to influence independence movements well into the twentieth century as peoples around the world sought to overthrow rulers and colonizers they came to regard as illegitimate.

At home, these words have inspired generations of American citizens to question the status quo and challenge authority. In what was probably his most influential speech, civil rights leader Martin Luther King Jr. drew extensively on the Declaration of

Independence, declaring: "I still have a dream. It is deeply rooted in the American dream. I have a dream that one day this nation will rise up, live out the true meaning of its creed: We hold these truths to be self-evident, that all men are created equal."

Just as Ron Ridenhour linked his protest to the country's founding backbone, King grounded political protest for the rights of Black Americans in the nation's original principles. What King and Ridenhour both understood was that the costs of dissent were necessary to advance the values embodied in the founding documents of their nation. In both cases, they were willing to pay a high price—from loathing to assassination—to ensure the country lived up to its creed.

PUNISHING MORAL REBELS

Certain truths may be self-evident, but the value of dissent is not one of them. It turns out that the merits of critics and the righteousness of rebels are in the eye of the beholder. It is easy when one is on the outside of a situation or looking back from the vantage of history to hold dissenters and whistleblowers in high esteem, even to regard them as heroes. But these people may seem something else entirely when one is faced with them in the present. In real life and in our own groups, they are often troublemakers, rabble-rousers, deviants, freaks, and all-around pains in the neck.

Americans now celebrate a national holiday in honor of Martin Luther King Jr. during which politicians, companies, and public figures of all kinds pay homage to his words and legacy. By 2011, MLK was almost universally perceived as a hero, and his national favorability rating was 94 percent. But during the civil rights era itself, opinions of MLK were sharply divided. In 1966, three years after he delivered his "I Have a Dream" speech, only 33 percent of Americans saw him as a positive figure.[4]

The fact is that in the present, people are often uncomfortable with "moral rebels"—people who live up to their values in the face of significant obstacles.

Benoît Monin and his colleagues have studied the mixed responses people often have to individuals doing the right thing.[5] In one experiment, for example, people learned about a prior participant who had been asked to write and record a speech in which she would have to publicly express an opinion that was contrary to her personal beliefs. Participants then had the chance to listen to what the earlier participant had recorded. One set of participants heard someone obediently doing the experimenter's bidding, articulating views that were not her own. However, another set of participants instead heard someone refusing to go along, disavowing any intention of saying things that she did not believe.

An act of agreeable obedience on the one hand and an act of principled disobedience on the other. If you were a participant yourself, which of these people would you have more respect for? If you are anything like us, you quite confidently assume that you would prefer the principled rebel.

But would you? Would we?

What we have not told you was that before they learned about anyone else, half of the participants in each of the conditions had also been asked to write and record their own speeches, and these participants had, to a person, complied with the experimenter's request to express an opinion with which they disagreed. The other half of the participants had received no such request and were thus simply uninvolved observers of another person's obedience or disobedience.

The uninvolved observers liked and respected the person they heard being rebellious more than the person they heard being obedient. They were impressed by someone willing to stand up for what she believed. If you came to the same conclusion, it is likely because you, the reader, were uninvolved.

But for those participants who had themselves been obedient, the pattern was completely reversed. They liked and respected the obedient speech giver more than the rebellious refuser.

In subsequent experiments, people learned about someone who had refused to complete a task on the grounds that it was probably racist. Critically, participants again learned about the rebel after they either had or had not completed the potentially racist task themselves. When asked to name a trait that they thought described this rebellious fellow subject, uninvolved observers (whose own behavior was not at stake) said that the moral rebel who had refused to complete the racist task was "strong-minded," "independent," "decisive," or "fair-minded." But participants who had already done the task themselves described the same rebel as "self-righteous," "defensive," "easily offended," or "confused." Why the difference?

From a distance, we admire moral rebels. But when they shake our belief that *we* are inherently good and virtuous people ourselves, it alters our perspective. In these instances, moral rebels make us look bad to ourselves and others, and we fear these more virtuous individuals will judge us negatively.

Who among us has not seen or heard about someone behaving unethically or immorally under pressure—perhaps cheating clients because the boss demanded it or bullying a coworker because everyone found it funny—and thought, *I would never do that!* And yet, at least some of the time, many of us do go along with things that we disagree with. By disobeying while others remain compliant, rebels expose the fact that many people often do not do the right thing when faced with a moral quandary. People do not acknowledge or maybe even realize their limitations until someone more courageous makes them aware of their own moral frailty. *Self-righteous jerk!* they think.

It turns out that people do not necessarily appreciate do-gooders, even when they are objectively doing good for their groups. It is not surprising that people react negatively to freeloaders, the sort of people who contribute little to a difficult group project but take plenty of credit when the project is successful or the kind who avoid paying taxes but draw heavily on government services. What is more startling, however, is that people can be just as negative toward highly generous group members.

Researchers Craig Parks and Asako Stone looked at people's responses to individuals who contributed a lot to a group resource but took little from it for themselves.[6] They found that when offered the opportunity to get rid of some group members, people were just as eager to expel these generous individuals as they were to kick out selfish ones!

When the researchers asked people why they reacted this way, some said that it was because the generous group member made them look bad by comparison. But a second type of explanation also emerged, one grounded in the sense that the generous person was breaking with group norms. Participants wrote, "It's strange for someone to keep giving and not take much in return. If you give a lot you should use a lot." And: "I probably would have been okay with him if I hadn't seen everyone else's choices and saw he was so different. He's too different from the rest of us."

In the scientific literature on how people respond to dissenters, rebels, and critics, it turns out there are a variety of things that trigger negative reactions. The thread that unites them is that they threaten people's identities. Sometimes, as with the moral rebels we discussed above, the threat is to group members' personal sense of self, but very often it is to their social identities and to what they believe are the interests and norms of the group.

People defend their group norms because these norms define them and help coordinate action; they get everyone on the same page. For this reason, deviants tend to be rejected more strongly in smaller groups, where they might do more damage to norms or dilute a consensus.[7]

Norm violators are judged particularly harshly when their actions blur the boundaries between groups, muddying the distinctions that members like to uphold between "us" and "them." Groups also tend not to appreciate deviance or dissent when they are under the pressure of a deadline or are embroiled in competition with an out-group.[8] A little divergence can be a healthy thing, but this is not the moment! When the group is at war, it's time to keep your mouth shut and rally around the flag. You are either with us or against us!

But groups that quash dissent are playing a dangerous game. Over time, embracing a diversity of opinions and listening to criticism is necessary for groups to flourish in the face of new challenges and adversity. Groups and organizations that demand too cultlike a conformity, like the ones we discussed in chapter 3, are often doomed to failure, sooner or later.

WHY WE NEED DISSENT

To properly understand the merits of dissent, criticism, and rebellion, it is clear we can't entirely rely on the opinions of people in the immediate situation. Fortunately, there is a sizable scientific literature on both the virtues and the downsides of dissent.

Charlan Nemeth, professor and author of the book *In Defense of Troublemakers,* has devoted much of her career to investigating the effects of dissent. She argues that the real benefits of dissenters come less from the ideas they espouse or suggestions they make than from the ways they change how the rest of us think.[9]

When people are exposed to popularly held ideas, their thinking tends to be lazy and narrow, focused on whether or not the majority view is correct. But when they hear a minority point of view, a rarer perspective, their thinking expands. They start to ponder why anyone would endorse that idea. Truth be told, they often start to argue against it, but in doing so they are forced to cast a wider net of thought, considering and perhaps even questioning their own assumptions.

This is critical because this is how dissent can improve innovation, creativity, and group decision-making. Dissent is effective because it changes the ways that other people think. This means that dissenters do not actually have to be right to benefit the group—they just have to speak up enough to get others thinking. Their mere presence can spark more divergent thought and open up space for others to express alternative views.

To measure the impact of dissent, researchers at the University of Michigan experimentally manipulated the presence or absence of dissenters in teams of students working together during the course of a semester.[10] Over ten weeks, twenty-eight teams engaged in problem-solving tasks and were evaluated on the originality of their solutions. The stakes were quite high for the students, as these problems were worth 40 percent of their final grades.

In half of the teams, one of the five members had, unbeknownst to the rest, been recruited by the research team to serve as a dissenter. This allowed the researchers to determine if the inclusion of a single dissenter within the team would improve performance or just create conflict and slow the team down.

The researchers did not blindly select these rebels. They needed people to whom divergence came reasonably naturally and who would be comfortable expressing disagreement. Thus, the fourteen dissenters were people who had, on a prior questionnaire, endorsed statements like "I expect to take risks with regard to expressing my ideas in my group" and "I value novelty in human behavior." The researchers provided some training, encouraging these students to be consistent and persistent when they dissented but not to appear rigid. They also asked them to express disagreement with their groups only when they really disagreed.

At the end of the semester, the results came in.

Adding a single dissenter to a small group paid off in several ways. Teams that were randomly assigned to include a dissenter performed better than those without. Their work was evaluated as more original by objective outside experts. Even the students working with dissenters noticed a difference. When they considered their own groups' patterns of thinking, they rated them as more divergent than students in groups without dissenters.

Similar processes play out in companies and organizations. In a study of seven Fortune 500 companies, organizational researchers used detailed case studies to examine how top leadership teams functioned at two points in time: during periods when they were successful and periods when they were widely perceived to be failing to satisfy key stakeholders.[11] The dynamics of the leadership teams were dramatically different during periods of success and failure.

The importance of shared identity was clearly associated with the successful periods. In these times, leadership teams appeared to have stronger feelings of "common fate," were more committed to solving group problems, showed more team spirit, and were more focused on shared goals.

Critically, these organizations also encouraged more dissent in private meetings and members were more open and candid with one another during successful periods. This reveals that dissent can flourish along with a strong sense of shared identity and a feeling of team spirit. In fact, those factors seem to be important parts of the recipe for group success in both the lab and the real world.

Research suggests that dissent is most likely to be effective when it is persistent and consistent. In the classic film *Twelve Angry Men*, starring Henry Fonda, a jury considers the guilt or innocence of an eighteen-year-old man accused of killing his father. The evidence seems clear and in an initial secret ballot, eleven of the twelve jurors are ready to vote guilty. One juror wants to wrap things up quickly because he has tickets to a baseball game.

Only one—juror number eight—thinks that the accused man might be innocent and that the evidence is not as solid as it seems.

Over the course of the next few hours, his observations and doubts slowly begin to change the minds of the other jurors, who themselves start to question the evidence. There are holdouts at first. But eventually the last proponent of a guilty verdict gives in. The jurors unanimously declare the young man not guilty.

The film is a rousing tale about the duty of dissent and about how a single, persistent skeptic can change the minds of others and alter the course of justice. More generally, it is the willingness of dissenters to stand their ground in the face of opposition that causes others to think more carefully. *This person must really believe what they are saying,* we think. *Why is that?*

As with everything involving human beings, however, the full story of dissent is a complicated one. Dissent does not have uniformly positive consequences for groups, and across studies the findings are mixed. In a recent meta-analysis, Codou Samba and colleagues found that *strategic dissent* among top management teams was associated with lower-quality decisions and lower performance.[12] This happened because it seemed to worsen relationships among team members and actually reduced their careful consideration of information.

Importantly, however, what these researchers refer to as *strategic dissent* reflects not just disagreement about how a group or organization should go about achieving its goals but about what those very goals should be. In the case of leadership teams, this conflict reflects a fracturing at the top of an organization about what they are trying to achieve and potentially who they are. As Samba and colleagues put it, "Strategic dissent does not so much capture diversity of information and insights that can be fruitfully integrated, but instead represents conflicting goals and preferences that members have a vested interest in defending. Strategic dissent, thus, disrupts information elaboration because managers are motivated to defend their positions rather than engage in an open-minded search and analysis."[13]

During their successful periods, the seven Fortune 500 companies mentioned earlier had elevated levels of dissent, but they also had palpable team spirit and were focused on shared goals. In the context of a clearly shared identity, dissent is beneficial. For teams that lack a shared identity or whose identity is seriously called into question, dissent is more challenging and difficult and may not always be associated immediately with better decisions or performance.

This is not to say that these disagreements are unimportant. Sometimes it is vital that groups—whether at the top of a management hierarchy or in society more broadly—debate and overhaul their goals, fundamentally reshaping who they are and what they stand for. But this process is unlikely to be easy.

To capitalize on the potential benefits of dissent, groups have to clear two hurdles: they have to have members willing to express divergent views, and the other members have to be able and willing to listen with curiosity rather than defensiveness. Both of these responses are grounded in strong and secure identities.

ARE PEOPLE SHEEPLE?

Although dissent, deviance, criticism, and rabble-rousing are clearly important, scientists have sunk much more of their time and energy into understanding their flip sides: conformity, compliance, and obedience. Psychologists' "conformist" focus on conformity can be traced to two key events in the discipline's history.

One was the conformity experiments conducted by Solomon Asch in which people went along with the erroneous judgments of other people despite the evidence of their own eyes.[14] As we described in chapter 2, participants in these studies were given an exceedingly easy visual task to solve: identifying which of several lines were the same in length. Everyone could do the task just fine until people answering ahead of them started to give wrong answers. Suddenly participants were confronted with pressure to conform, which they gave into about a third of the time, answering the questions incorrectly themselves to go along with the crowd.

The second major event was a series of studies conducted a few years later by Yale psychologist Stanley Milgram.[15] Milgram expanded on Asch's conformity findings by examining how a single powerful person might shape behavior when the stakes were much higher than estimating lines.

He recruited residents of New Haven, Connecticut, for an experiment on how punishment affects learning. Participants arrived at Yale University in pairs and were met by an experimenter in a lab coat. Just like Asch, Milgram staged the situation so that only one member of each pair was there as a true subject—the other was secretly working for the research team. The real participants were all assigned to be the "teacher" in the experiment; they were told they would be testing the memory of a partner who was assigned to be the "learner."

The teacher was asked to read lists of word pairs to the learner, who then had to recite them back. The twist was that every time the learner made a mistake, the teacher had to deliver an escalating electric shock as punishment for the error. The shocks started small at fifteen volts but increased by fifteen volts with every mistake. As the study progressed and the learner made more errors, the required voltages were labeled with increasingly forbidding warnings: INTENSE SHOCK, DANGER SEVERE SHOCK, and finally just XXX at 450 volts.

When these shocks were delivered by the teacher, the learner had been instructed to emit more and more intense complaints, expressions of pain, and requests to stop before falling ominously silent. If the teacher protested, the experimenter would respond firmly: "Please continue," "The experiment requires you to continue," "It is absolutely essential that you continue," and, finally, "You have absolutely no choice but to continue." In reality, of course, there were no shocks, and the whole scenario was an elaborate ruse.

Would you shock a complete stranger despite hearing him scream in agony or complain of heart problems? Most people say they would not.

Before conducting his experiment, Stanley Milgram asked a group of psychiatrists how they thought people would react when instructed to administer apparently dangerous shocks to a fellow participant. The clinicians' consensus was that only one person in a thousand would be fully compliant.

The experts were wildly wrong. In the standard version of the experiment, nearly two thirds of participants fully obeyed the instructions of the experimenter. A sizable majority of people delivered the maximum level of shock to an apparently unconscious learner simply because they had been instructed to do so by a man wearing a lab coat.

In neither Asch's nor Milgram's studies were people happy about the situation they found themselves in. Asch's participants appeared confused as they tried to figure out what on earth was going on. *How can everyone else be mistaken? Is something wrong with my eyes?* Many of Milgram's participants questioned the experimenter. *Are you sure? Shouldn't we check on him?* To which the experimenter responded implacably, "Please continue, the experiment must go on." And many of them did go on to the very end, shocking an apparently helpless man in the room next door over and over again.

Initially, the results of these studies were hugely surprising and provocative to people. They illuminated aspects of human behavior that few expected. Many people saw parallels between Milgram's experiments and the atrocities of the Holocaust. But ideas change, and these findings quickly went from shocking revelations to common wisdom, at least among social scientists. The lessons from Asch and Milgram seemed clear. People are highly conformist; they are sheeplike in the face of even mild pressure from peers. People are also blindly obedient to authority, and this unthinking compliance might lead them to participate in great evil.

In textbooks and popular-psychology books, these are often still the lessons drawn from these studies. But expert understanding of these issues has continued to evolve, and social scientists interpret them differently today. The lessons of these classic studies are more nuanced and complex—and might even surprise people who learned about these studies long ago. In each case, the story has much more to do with social identities than was previously understood.

WE'RE NOT SHEEP AFTER ALL

As graduate students at the University of Toronto, the two of us spent many happy hours perusing secondhand bookstores in the Annex, a bustling neighborhood adjoining the downtown campus. Procrastinating on our dissertation work, we could convince ourselves that we were being productive by diligently checking out the psychology section in each store. Idly gazing at the shelves one day, Dom spotted a copy of *Obedience to Authority*, the book in which Stanley Milgram comprehensively described his obedience studies, a steal at $6.99. He snapped it up.

It is often safe to assume that the more famous a piece of research is, the less likely it is that people have actually read the original account. Over a million students take an introduction to psychology class each year, and most of them learn the textbook version of Milgram's studies. After enough retellings, the studies become like myths—the key findings are amplified while critical details and context are slowly lost to future generations.

Students also learn that Milgram's research was ethically dubious because it deceived people into behaving badly and that nothing like it would be permitted today. What need, then, is there to dust off the primary source? With a million other things to read, who has the time?

Still procrastinating, however, Dom found the time and it led him to a fascinating new discovery.[16] Milgram ran a variety of different obedience studies. In each study, he manipulated a different feature of the situation to try to figure out what factors affected rates of obedience. He found that increasing the physical closeness of the person being shocked decreased obedience. He found that women responded in much the same way as men. He also found that having the experimenter issue instructions over the telephone reduced obedience, although some participants felt the need to lie and tell the absent experimenter that they had continued to deliver shocks to the hapless learner.

Milgram's book provided the raw data for many of these studies. A table indicated the number of people who had stopped participating at every voltage point, from 15 volts all the way up to 450. As Dom read about each variant of the study, his eyes were increasingly drawn to these data and, in particular, to the disobedient participants. He was fascinated by those people who had withdrawn before they reached the final 450-volt shock—the people who had dissented in the face of a cruel authority figure. Who were these moral rebels?

To Dom's surprise, he began to see a pattern to this disobedience. Milgram's book made no mention of this pattern, and Dom had not heard anyone talk about it before. Were his eyes deceiving him? It took a matter of minutes to enter data from several of Milgram's studies into a spreadsheet and plot them on a graph. He turned to Jay, seated right behind him in their office, and asked, "Am I seeing this right?"

In each experiment, there were twenty-nine points in time at which a participant could disobey the experimenter, ranging from 15 volts on the very first trial to 435 volts on the penultimate one. Yet when Dominic looked at the data closely, the points at which

217

THE POWER OF US

participants had actually disobeyed were not uniformly or randomly arrayed across these possibilities. Rather, disobedience seemed to peak at particular times and at one especially: a key moment of truth seemed to have occurred when it was time to deliver a shock of 150 volts.

What was so special about 150 volts? Why was this point in the study different from 135 volts or 165 volts? Dominic scrambled back to find the original methods to figure it out.

As we noted earlier, the learner in Milgram's studies followed a script, uttering an escalating series of complaints, pleas, and expressions of pain to every participant as the shocks increased. His expressions of pain grew in intensity until he eventually fell silent.

But the 150-volt point was qualitatively different. It was the first (but not the last) time at which the learner asked specifically to be released from the experiment. He shouted, "Experimenter, get me out of here! I won't be in the experiment anymore! I refuse to go on!"

This first request was a turning point. Participants faced a crucial choice: either they listened to and complied with the wishes of the learner or they obeyed the instructions of the experimenter, in which case they would probably continue all the way to the end.

Similar requests by the learner as the study progressed did not have this same effect. It was the first one that really mattered. And although the learner's expressions of pain continued to grow as the shocks increased, rates of disobedience were unaffected, suggesting that the decision to stop shocking a fellow human being was not driven by empathic reactions to their suffering. Something else was going on.

So what did drive their decisions? A recent analysis by Steve Reicher, Alex Haslam, and Joanne Smith suggests that experiencing a sense of shared identity, either with the experimenter or with the learner, likely played a key role in participants' choices.[17] And it was at the 150-volt mark that participants had to choose a side: Whose team were they on, the experimenter's or the learner's?

The inability to directly replicate Milgram's research has stymied many an investigation, but this trio of researchers came up with a clever workaround. Half a century after the original research, they told participants, including a group of expert psychologists and a group of undergraduates, about different versions of Milgram's experiments. For each variant of the experiment, they asked these participants to rate how much they thought they would identify with the scientist and scientific community versus the learner as a member of the general public.

People thought that they would identify more with the experimenter and less with the learner in some variants of Milgram's studies, such as when the learner was physically remote. For other versions, they thought the opposite, such as when the experimenter was literally phoning it in.

Taking these current-day ratings of identification, the researchers tested whether they could predict what the actual, real participants in the original experiments had done back in the 1960s. And they could! Current-day participants' beliefs that they would identify with the experimenter strongly predicted greater obedience in the original Milgram experiments conducted five decades earlier. In contrast, their beliefs that they would identify with the learner strongly predicted less obedience in the original studies.

Obedience and disobedience, then, both seem to be a matter of identity. Whose side are you on? Are you with the scientist in the lab coat, with all that he represents about knowledge, progress, and expertise? Or are you with the member of the public, with all the rights of a fellow citizen? Once people made this decision, it shaped their willingness to engage in dissent or continue along the path to cruelty.

RATIONAL CONFORMITY AND IRRATIONAL DISSENT

Shortly after Dom published his analysis of Milgram's obedience data, he met Bert Hodges. Hodges and his colleagues had just flipped the script on Solomon Asch's famous line-perception experiments.[18] In the original studies in the 1950s, participants clearly saw the correct answers on a visual task but heard everyone else get them wrong, which led them to conform. In this new version, the study was set up so that participants could hear other people's answers, but they could not clearly see the task themselves. Participants had to identify words projected onto a screen at the front of the room, but they were seated in such a way that it was difficult to make out the right answer. As in Asch's studies, other participants—who could clearly see the words—responded first.

Imagine yourself in the shoes of the participant. Through no fault of your own, you cannot see well enough to properly complete the task. Fortunately, however, other people can and they are answering ahead of you. What would you do? While conforming to obviously incorrect answers in Asch's original study was uncomfortable, here, conforming to other people's presumably correct answers would make perfect sense. In good conscience, you can sit back, relax, and go along with the crowd.

And that is what participants did about two-thirds of the time. But on the other trials, they did something counterintuitive: they guessed and made up an answer that was almost certainly wrong. Approximately one-third of the time, people chose not to draw upon the information they received from more knowledgeable others. Strikingly, this proportion of "irrational" nonconformist behavior was almost the same as the proportion of "irrational" conformist behavior in the original study, which also occurred about one-third of the time.

But the behaviors of people in both Asch's original and the

inverted conformity studies are irrational only if we assume that people are motivated by one goal and one goal alone: the desire to be accurate. Clearly they are not. Asch's original participants were also motivated by the goal of fitting in, being liked and accepted by others. But this goal too was not so all-consuming that people conformed all of the time.

People possess numerous goals. They are almost always trying to accomplish more than one thing at a time, and the actions they choose to take often reflect an attempt to balance among them. When you are with other people, you strive to be a good social partner, and when you are in a group, you aim to be a solid, contributing, and useful member. There are multiple ways to do this. Being accurate and providing correct information is important. But so is establishing friendly and trusting relationships, and so is telling the truth about who you are, in a broader sense than simply giving the objectively right answer.

Everyone has been in this situation. You are sitting with friends, coworkers, or family members, and they all agree about something you know is utterly ridiculous. "*Cats* is a great movie!" "Eggnog is delicious and not a bit cloying!" "Cabbots are what happens when a cat mates with a rabbit—and they really exist!" But as the righteous urge to correct your compatriots bubbles up, you push it back down. *Let's keep the peace,* you think. You are having a good time; you can set the record straight later. Your broader truth is *I am here, I am one of you, and I want to make this thing with all of you work.*

This is what participants in Asch's original experiments were doing: balancing between goals. They were walking a tightrope between giving accurate answers that put them at odds with others and giving accommodating responses that signaled a willingness to play along to maintain good standing in the group. In the inverted version of the experiment, a different tightrope act took place. Here, people sought to balance between being accurate—which in this case meant mirroring the responses of others—and making

221

unique contributions to the group. As much as standing out from the crowd can be uncomfortable, we do not like to feel that we are mindlessly copying others all of the time either. By diverging once in a while, participants could maintain a degree of independence and also signal to others that they were not to be relied on as good sources of information, a useful acknowledgment when their view was obscured.

These studies reveal some critical lessons about human nature. First, people are not blindly obedient to authorities. Resistance and dissent are as much a part of human nature as conformity. Instead, what matters is who we identify with: are we aligned with those in positions of authority or with more ordinary people whose wishes and rights we think should be heard and taken into account?

Second, people are not inevitably sheeplike in the face of pressure from their peers. We do, it is true, frequently conform to the behavior of others, and for good reasons. But we also often have good reasons not to conform. When we choose to deviate, it is usually not because we do not care what others think or because we want to be difficult. We usually deviate because we want to be useful to our groups.

Groups tend to make better decisions when people can express divergent views. A little bit of dissent can inject a vital piece of new information, broaden people's thinking, or make it more comfortable for others to speak up. And sometimes dissent simply causes us to reassess assumptions one more time, confirming with a bit more confidence that we are on the right track.

THE CHOICES WE FACE

So when will people do this important work? And how can groups, whether they are neighborhood coalitions, work organizations, or even nation-states, foster healthy levels of dissent?

Imagine a few scenarios. You are a border guard and you have noticed a tendency among your coworkers to question certain types of travelers more aggressively than others. Or you work for a midsize company and it is common practice for employees on your team to spend a couple of hours a day on social media instead of doing their jobs. Or you work for a small start-up firm where everyone from the boss on down competes to be the most hardworking, putting in very long days, coming in on weekends, and boasting about how busy they are. Or perhaps you are a member of a volunteer organization where folks are not shy about expressing their disdain for people who disagree with them politically, even though you know there are such people working diligently—and silently—among you.

To figure out what you might do in these sorts of situations, we can ask a series of questions. The first is quite simple: *Do you disagree with the norm or are you okay with it?* Perhaps you have never thought about it before—never asked yourself, for example, whether paying people to surf social media is a good use of your company's resources. Or you have thought about the norm, but you do not have a problem with it. Some types of people should, you might believe, be questioned more intensively than others at the border. Or if people want to work long hours at your start-up firm, fine—it is up to them. If you do not disagree with the norm, you are probably not going to turn around and question it. If you do disagree, you might.

But then we need to ask a second question: *How much do you identify with the group?*[19] Identification matters because it influences whose interests you are motivated to pursue. Even at the best of times, dissent is difficult; remember how people react to moral rebels. Dissent might not be worth the trouble unless you deeply care about the group, your fellow members, and your collective future.

Let's say you are weakly identified with the group. In other words, you disagree with a norm in a group that you don't particularly care for. Faced with this situation, do you invest your time and energy in dissenting? Do you expose yourself to the social flak that almost inevitably comes along with it? Probably not. In this case, you are quite likely to disengage further from the group. You might express your opinion to your outside friends, but not in the hope of changing anyone's mind or making the group a better place. Depending on the gravity of your conflict with the norm, you might even quit entirely. Bye, suckers!

But what if this is a group that you do care deeply about? In this case, dissent might just be worth it. You are invested in the group and want it to succeed. You want it to be a well-regarded group, a successful group, an ethical and moral group. In this case, you *might* be motivated to challenge your group to try to change it for the better.

You worry that treating some travelers differently as they cross the border will undermine the public's trust in border agents, undercut your effectiveness, or reduce morale. You think that some of your team's recent performance woes could be solved if people focused a bit more on their jobs and less on posting selfies to Instagram or polishing their résumés on LinkedIn. You notice that the competitive "Who works the hardest?" culture at your start-up is burning out good people and weeding out certain kinds of folks, especially women with kids. You worry that this culture is not sustainable in the long run and undercuts your ability to retain the best talent. Or within your highly dedicated volunteer organization, you believe it is important as a matter of principle that people who think differently should nevertheless be treated with respect.

When you see a problem and care about the group, whether you are likely to actually dissent depends on the answer to a third question: *What do you expect the consequences of dissent to be?* There are two types of potential consequences that matter: those affecting you as an individual and those affecting the group as a whole.

Consequences for the individual are important. As we have seen, deviance is often met with negative reactions, reactions that can sting all the more when they come from close compatriots in a beloved group. Your devotion to the group may be enough for you to risk sacrificing the goodwill and acceptance of others, but as the severity of personal sanctions increases, so too will your discomfort and disinclination to speak out. Consequences for the group really start to matter now. If you think that, despite a negative reception, your dissent has a reasonably good chance of changing the group—of actually making things better—you might still go for it. But if you sense that achieving change is unlikely or impossible, dissenting may seem, quite simply, not worth it. This is the cost-benefit analysis of dissent.

We can draw the route to your likely decision through a series of forking paths. First fork: Do you disagree with the norm? Second fork: Are you strongly identified with the group? Third fork: Do the potential benefits of dissent outweigh the potential costs? If the answer to all of these questions is yes, you are quite likely to dissent.

INSPIRING DISSENT

We celebrate dissenters and critics as heroes in the abstract or when we can hold them at a distance. We also like to think of ourselves as the kind of people who would bravely speak out when they notice wrongdoing or think there is a better way of accomplishing things. But research suggests that when confronted with actual dissenters—with moral rebels—people are often discomfited and react by derogating or rejecting them. And when they encounter substantive disagreements with their groups, people often remain silent or distance themselves rather than summoning the courage to try to change things for the better.

If group members or leaders want to do something about this state of affairs, want to create cultures where people speak up when something is wrong, what should they do? If we hope to foster groups in which people are free to express their perspectives and have the capacity to learn from divergent views, how could we go about it?

In some of our research we have focused on the first fork in the road by simply asking people to think about ways in which norms might be harmful to their groups.[20] Once we got people to think about these problems, strongly identified members were more willing to express dissenting views. In fact, they were more willing to dissent than both weakly identified members *and* strongly identified members who had thought about how a norm was harmful to themselves personally.

The key to dissent was that they saw the harm to a group that they cared about.

We have also tested more subtle ways of prompting people to think critically about what their groups are up to.[21] In particular, getting people to think more abstractly seems to open them up to divergent thoughts about group behavior. There are different ways of getting people to think abstractly, but a common one is to encourage longer-term as opposed to shorter-term thinking. When we think in the short term, we focus on immediate needs and goals. Often this involves a sense of urgency—*We just need to get this done*—and the feeling that now is not the time to raise questions or doubts.

When we think in the longer term, however, we become more attentive to the possibility of change and improvement. Thinking five or ten years down the road raises the question "Do we still want to be doing this then?" Will we be able to make the transition from start-up to profitable company if we keep burning people out with crazy work hours? Will today's national security concerns be the same tomorrow and, if not, how will we repair relations with communities if we damage them with disparate treatment now? If we cannot get employees to spend less time online and more time doing their jobs, will we even exist in five years? Is political bias within our volunteer organization driving away dedicated contributors and will it undermine our credibility?

To investigate the role of time in dissent, we studied supporters of the Republican Party and their willingness to challenge popular positions within their party.[22] In one case, for example, we asked people whether they would be willing to publicly express concern about the Republican Party's opposition to the Affordable Care Act, also known as Obamacare.

Three things mattered in terms of their willingness to speak out. First, as we have discussed, they had to disagree with the standard party position—and some did. Second, they had to be strongly identified with the Republican Party. And third, they had to be worried about the *future* consequences for the Republican Party itself. In this case, they had to be concerned that opposition to publicly funded health care would hurt the party's prospects in future elections. When these three things lined up, we observed greater willingness to dissent.

To aspiring change agents, we would suggest a couple of things. The first is that it is okay to be weakly identified with a group. Not every group you are a part of is necessarily worth identifying with. We think, for example, that it was a good thing when participants in Milgram's experiments did not identify with the experimenter. This lack of identification with authority and identification with the learner instead led people to do the right thing and disobey harmful instructions.

Second, in order to be in a position to dissent at all, you have to be able to think critically about what your group is doing. You have to experience some sort of disagreement. This sounds simple, but it is not. If everyone spends time on social media at work, it becomes a default or habit. It is just how things are done, and you might never give it a second thought. If everyone works insane hours, it might not seem insane; it's just the reality of how we work. By the time these norms become problematic, many people within the group have rationalized and internalized them, thinking that if they do not work long hours, the company will go bankrupt or the team will surely fail.

THE POWER OF US

Sometimes bad patterns develop and worsen with the same logic that led Milgram's participants to shock someone (or so they believed) with 450 volts. A 15-volt shock does not seem too bad. People can rationalize it and comfortably up the voltage to 30 volts, then 45 volts, and so on. Each small step makes the next step easier. Once they get past the 150-volt mark, they are likely to just continue going all the way up to 450 volts. What had once seemed unthinkable becomes routine.

When the potential downsides to group norms are pointed out, however, many people can immediately see them, although they may not have noticed them spontaneously themselves. To do so requires a broadening of focus from the immediate present or task to the future or the larger meaning of things. This may be why dissent tends to be greater among people who score higher on the personality trait of openness to experience.[23] People who are highly open tend to think about things in more creative and abstract ways, making more connections between disparate thoughts. They also tend to seek out more unique experiences, which may expose them to divergent perspectives.

If you are in a group with which you are weakly identified, it is worth paying attention when you observe yourself conforming in ways that make you uncomfortable. You do not usually feel like you have to work on weekends, but you do when the regional manager is in town. You generally do not make fun of others who disagree with you politically, but somehow you find yourself doing so in the company of your colleagues. These shifts in behavior are a signal that you are not indifferent to the norm; that, in fact, you might have a problem with it. Feeling compelled to change your actions from what you would normally do can be a sign that something is amiss.

Hopefully, though, you get to spend most of your time in groups that you care about and identify with. Here, you are motivated to do what you believe is in the group's best interests and you want to do right by the group. But what is in the group's best interests? And what does it mean to do right by the group? Those are the key questions.

If, as a leader, you want to encourage people to dissent more often when they see a problem and avoid a culture of groupthink, your levers reside at the forks in the decision-making road we have described. People need to think critically enough to experience disagreement. They need to identify strongly with the group and care enough to speak up. And, of course, people need to think that the consequences of dissent make it worthwhile. If the likely costs are too high or the likely benefits are too low, dissent is unlikely.

Get people thinking longer term about what your group is trying to do. In organizations, if the boss is interested predominantly in short-term outcomes or if management jumps from immediate crisis to immediate crisis, employees will adopt the same focus. They will feel they have to. However, if every once in a while, leaders stop to ask about longer-term consequences or about where people want to be in ten years, others will feel licensed to think in that way as well. An obsession with quarterly returns might be one of the most powerful incentives promoting groupthink and undercutting dissent—and a similar dynamic may affect politicians stuck in perpetual election cycles.

Leaders should be especially attentive to the signals they send about the costs of dissent. As much as people can be reluctant to deviate from peers, the pressure to keep one's mouth shut is often greater in hierarchical situations and when the boss is around. People are more willing to speak up in groups and organizations when they believe that offering divergent ideas and opinions is not risky and especially if it is explicitly valued. Leaders at all levels play a key role in creating these feelings of "psychological safety."[24]

Organizational psychologist Amy Edmondson studied how leaders promoted psychological safety in cardiac operating teams as they learned a new way of conducting heart surgery.[25] This new surgical

229

technique required that these teams, composed of surgeons, anes-thesiologists, nurses, and technicians, work as perfectly coordinated units despite big differences in training, disciplinary backgrounds, and certainly status. And the stakes were incredibly high—their ability to communicate was literally a matter of life and death.

She observed that surgical teams where members had a voice and felt comfortable speaking up were more successful at adopting the new lifesaving technique. She found that some surgeons, the team leaders, were better at creating this type of psychological safety than others. The leaders of more successful teams invested more energy communicating the importance of their mission—learning the new technique. But they also worked harder to reduce power disparities within their teams, trying to put everyone on something closer to an equal footing. When others had things to say, these leaders made sure to listen and take action. They took care to highlight the importance of every person's role, and they demonstrated humility by noting their own limitations. They also avoided overreacting to errors, often choosing to adapt and move on when a team member made a mistake rather than calling the individual out.

A similar pattern was observed at Google. They set out to deter-mine what factors made for the most effective teams.[26] They looked at 180 teams from across the company to identify skill sets or person-ality types that accounted for group success. Google is famous for crunching data and finding patterns—but there were virtually no patterns to be found. According to Abeer Dubey, one of the leaders of Project Aristotle (as the study was known): "We had lots of data, but there was nothing showing that a mix of specific personality types or skills or backgrounds made any difference. The 'who' part of the equation didn't seem to matter."

But one thing did predict team success. The research team at Google concluded that group dynamics were actually the key to team success. In particular, their data revealed that *psychological safety*, more than anything else, was critical to making a team effective. The best teams provided a supportive environment in which people could voice alternative perspectives without fear of negative consequences.

People often think that psychological safety means you cannot criticize at all. But what it actually means is quite the opposite—psychologically safe environments are ones in which people feel safe expressing divergent perspectives because debate is welcomed and embraced. These are groups where people can disagree respectfully and come back together the next day without hard feelings. They can challenge ideas and practices because all the members feel like they are working toward the same goals.

Smart leaders and organizations focus on cultivating environments where people feel psychologically safe and on reducing the costs associated with dissent. Some organizations have gone even further and found ways to reward constructive dissent. The American Foreign Service Association exemplifies this ethos. Every year, it gives four "Constructive Dissent Awards," cosponsored with the director general of the Foreign Service, to actively serving personnel. As the website states:

> The awards publicly recognize individuals who have demonstrated the intellectual courage to challenge the system from within, to question the status quo and take a stand, no matter the sensitivity of the issue or the consequences of their actions.[27]

By clearly recognizing the value of dissent for the institution—and, by proxy, the nation as a whole—the organization increases the rewards associated with taking these sorts of actions. It also helps that each award comes with a four-thousand-dollar prize on top of the recognition!

Of course, most of us are not in a position to create awards for constructive dissent. But we are still a crucial part of the equation simply as ordinary group members. How we react to divergent perspectives, whether we are willing to listen, and how we treat the person expressing a unique opinion shapes dissenters' willingness to carry on. It probably also affects the future behavior of other people who are paying attention to what happens. While our natural inclinations are often to resist counter-normative actions and actors, we know that these things are often good for our groups and that they frequently come from people who do, in fact, care.

So take a deep breath and, rather than jumping immediately to conclusions about nefarious motives, give dissenters, critics, and rebels a chance. There is a good possibility, as the American Foreign Service Association recognizes, that they intend to be constructive.

But ultimately, who cares what their motives are? As research on the effects of deviance and dissent shows, one of the major benefits of dissent is that it gets the rest of us thinking. The dissenter does not have to be right to invigorate our thinking and increase the chances that we will make better and more innovative decisions. Having a devil's advocate on your team could benefit everyone.

If we understand that dissent is good for our groups, we may be more receptive to it. But sometimes that might not be enough. You might be nodding along to our suggestions, but think back to the studies on moral rebels at the beginning of this chapter. People were resistant to others who deviated on matters of principle when they themselves had not done so because they felt it called into question their own wisdom and integrity. To avoid this threat to self-image, participants in these studies downplayed and disparaged the rebels, calling them "self-righteous" and "confused."

Thankfully, Benoît Monin and colleagues have found a potential antidote to this less-than-helpful reaction. They found that reminding participants of recent experiences in which they exhibited behaviors consistent with values that they held dear reduced the threat posed by a moral rebel.[28] This affirmation exercise reminded people that they often were, in fact, wise and good, and it seemed to free them to see the wisdom and goodness in others, even when they themselves may not have behaved as well as they could have in that particular moment.

Here is how Monin and colleagues affirmed their participants:

Please write about a recent experience in which you demonstrated a quality or value that is very important to you and which made you feel good about yourself. Examples might include (but are not limited to) artistic skills, sense of humor, social skills, spontaneity, athletic ability, musical talent, physical attractiveness, creativity, business skills, or romantic values.

You can try it now if you like or, better yet, the next time you do not want to hear what a troublemaker or rabble-rouser has to say. And with any luck, as time goes on, some of the experiences you will be proud to write about will include providing room for others to dissent and engaging in a bit of righteous rebellion yourself.

CHAPTER 9

LEADING EFFECTIVELY

When we think of leaders in action, a set of simple iconic images often comes to mind.

We might think of Jacinda Ardern, the prime minister of New Zealand, reacting to an earthquake during a live television interview. Talking about her country's highly effective response to the COVID-19 pandemic, Ardern remains cool and collected as the ground beneath her rattles and shakes. "We're just having a bit of an earthquake here, Ryan," she coolly tells the interviewer before assuring him that she is fine to carry on.[1]

We might picture Winston Churchill walking among the wreckage of demolished buildings, greeting Londoners as they sweep up rubble following a night of heavy German bombing.

We might imagine seamstress Rosa Parks quietly but firmly refusing to move to the back of a bus in racially segregated Montgomery, Alabama.

We might see Mahatma Gandhi leading a march of many thousands of Indian protesters hundreds of miles to the sea. Reaching at long last the shore, he stoops to pick up grains of salt, breaking the tax laws, which prohibit the Indian population from collecting or selling their own salt. A powerful yet nonviolent strike against a symbol of British imperial oppression.

We might also envision the famous photo of President Barack Obama, taken early in his first term, bending low in the Oval Office to let a little Black boy touch his hair. A moment earlier, Jacob Philadelphia, the five-year-old son of a staffer, had whispered, "I want to know if my hair is just like yours." "Why don't you touch it and see for yourself. Touch it, dude," Obama responded as he lowered his head for Jacob to reach.[2]

Leadership is a deeply complex phenomenon. Despite millennia of thinking about it, researchers have yet to fully answer even the most basic of questions: What makes some leaders effective while others fail? What drives some people to seek to lead? Why do other people consent to be led? How can leadership abilities be developed? What abilities are necessary? When are leaders a force for good, when are they a force for evil, and can evil leaders be thwarted?

In his wonderful book *Leading Minds,* psychologist Howard Gardner provides case studies of eminent twentieth-century leaders.[3] The eleven people whose lives and tactics, successes and failures he probes are a varied bunch. They range from scholarly and scientific leaders, like Margaret Mead and J. Robert Oppenheimer, through military, religious, and business leaders, to social and political leaders like Martin Luther King Jr., Margaret Thatcher, and Gandhi. Despite many striking differences between his subjects, Gardner draws out critical things they have in common. Fundamentally, he argues, what great leaders do, no matter their domain, is tell stories about identity:

> What links the eleven individuals...and the score of others from this century whose names could readily have been substituted for them, is the fact that they arrived at a story that worked for them and, ultimately, for others as well. They told stories—in so many words—about themselves and their groups, about where they were coming from and where they were headed, about what was to be feared, struggled against, and dreamed about.

But Gardner makes it clear that it is not enough simply to tell stories; leaders must embody them:

> Leaders...convey their stories by the kinds of lives they themselves lead and, through example, seek to inspire in their followers. The ways in which direct leaders conduct their lives—their embodiments—must be clearly perceptible by those they seek to influence.

Iconic moments of leadership, like the ones described above, are instances of embodiment. They are powerful because they capture an essence. But it is an essence not simply of the leaders themselves—their particular dynamism or brilliance or charisma—it is an essence of *us,* of the group as a whole. They are moments in which the actions of a leader exemplify something about who we are or perhaps who we aspire to be.

With her unflappable reaction to the earthquake, Jacinda Ardern carried forward the calm, collected, and collectively oriented style with which New Zealand had confronted a terrible terror attack in Christchurch in 2019 and then the COVID-19 pandemic.

Churchill striding amid the rubble signified British courage and resilience as the Brits—at the time, more or less alone—confronted Hitler's Germany.

Dignified and humble, Rosa Parks's simple act of refusal, for which she was arrested and charged with violating Alabama's segregation laws, started something that could not be stopped and became a powerful symbol of nonviolent resistance to racial injustice. At a rally a few days later, following the first organized boycott of buses in Montgomery, twenty-six-year-old Martin Luther King Jr. spoke. "Nobody," he said of Rosa Parks, "can doubt the boundless reach of her integrity. Nobody can doubt the height of her character....And just because she refused to get up, she was arrested. And you know, my friends, there comes a time when people get tired of being trampled over by the iron feet of oppression."[4] This was King's first political speech and a turning point in the struggle for civil rights and for the country.

Bending down to let a five-year-old boy touch his hair in the Oval Office, President Obama embodied the continuation of that struggle. Until then, Black children in America had never seen someone who looked like themselves in such high office. It was a moment in American history made possible by the accomplishments of the civil rights movement, when the very existence of a Black president afforded hope for continued progress toward a more just and equitable society.

Obama also embodied a certain American cool. "Touch it, dude."

Of all these leaders, Gandhi probably took the greatest care to ensure that he visibly embodied his story about Indian independence and nonviolent struggle. He took to wearing a loincloth of simple spun fabric, dramatizing his connection to the poor and initiating a movement to boycott the British-controlled fabric industry by encouraging Indians to spin their own. The spinning wheel became a symbol of the independence movement. So too did salt.

These snapshots are evocative because they show a leader embodying an identity, when the story he or she sought to tell about the group's identity was captured in a moment of authentic action.

Of course, for many of these examples, we know what happened next. We can see that a leader who unites the group around an identity today may fail to do so tomorrow. We can see that no leader's story tells the entire truth about a group. We can also see that no story goes uncontested. There are always competing visions about where we come from and where we are going, what we must fear, struggle against, and dream about. For this reason, leadership can be understood, in many ways, as a battle of stories.

WHAT IS LEADERSHIP?

Management guru and professor Henry Mintzberg points out that actually running a group involves a host of different tasks.[5] Sometimes you are a spokesperson, talking up the team to outside constituencies. Sometimes you are a monitor, scanning the environment for opportunities and threats to the group. Sometimes you are an entrepreneur, developing strategy in response to those opportunities and threats. Sometimes (perhaps too often) you are a disturbance handler, reacting to crises within and without, taking care of HR and PR problems alike. And at other times, you are a resource allocator and a negotiator, deciding who gets what or trying to work out mutually acceptable sets of outcomes.

So what is leadership? There are nearly as many definitions of the word as there are people who have written about it. But most scholars are willing to settle for Howard Gardner's definition: *leadership* is "the capacity of a person (or group of persons) to influence other people." President Harry Truman expressed much the same idea in more cynical terms. A leader is a person, he said, "who can persuade people to do what they don't want to do and like it."[6]

These broad definitions highlight the fact that leaders are as likely to be found on the local soccer field as they are in corporate boardrooms or political offices. Leaders need not hold a formal or high-level position. Indeed, in business, the greatest influence can come from a union steward or a rogue middle manager rather than the C-suite. On the soccer pitch, it can come from the midfielder rather than the coach.

For the past couple of decades, a large body of research has examined "transformational leadership." Transformational leaders exhibit a cluster of desirable characteristics.[7] They are ethical and committed to the well-being of their organizations, serving as models of integrity. They encourage people to establish ambitious goals and inspire them to do their best. They trust people to think critically and for themselves. And they support people emotionally as well as practically. Unsurprisingly, people enjoy having transformational leaders, and this style is associated with good performance among individual workers, teams, and organizations.

No one could doubt that transformational leadership is a good thing. However, when researchers Frank Wang and Jane Howell looked at studies on transformational leadership in the workplace, they noticed that they tended to conflate two types of behaviors.[8] Some aspects of transformational leadership focus on how leaders treat followers as individuals, showing concern about their professional development and career progression, for example. These are the sorts of things that make for a good boss, the sense that this is a person who knows who you are, recognizes your accomplishments, and cares about your aspirations. Other aspects of transformational leadership, however, focus on group-oriented activities, such as sharing a vision for a team and building solidarity around a common sense of purpose.

They reasoned that these different types of behaviors might foster two different kinds of identity. *Individually oriented leadership* might create relational identities in which individuals feel a personalized bond with a leader—feeling cared for and also caring about their leader. *Group-oriented leadership* activities, however, might create a strong social identity—feelings of solidarity and a shared sense of purpose for the group as a whole.

Studying a large Canadian company, Wang and Howell found that employees with more individually focused managers, the type who communicated high expectations and developed their skills, felt more personally identified with their leaders. These feelings of identification with the leader predicted better individual performance on the job and feelings of empowerment.

But employees who had more group-focused managers, the type who communicated a vision and spent time building collective camaraderie, felt more identified with their work teams. These teams also showed higher levels of performance as a group and felt more effective. Importantly, stronger team-based social identities were associated with better performance by individual team members as well.

Effective leaders engage in both individual and collective forms of transformational leadership. Both are things people want to see in managers and supervisors, not to mention coaches and mentors. There are myriad books and articles about leadership that focus on building strong relationships, providing effective feedback, developing strategies, allocating resources, and handling HR issues. Our approach is different—we will focus on the ways leaders influence others by managing their social identities.

Leaders often seek to influence their followers' feelings of identification and the content of their social identities; that is, their conceptions of "who we are." But ultimately, whether or not the identity stories told by leaders are embraced lies in the hands of the followers.

LEADERS' STORIES

Mary Robinson was elected the first female president of Ireland in 1990. The election of a woman was a sudden, startling change for the nation, caused at least in part by the self-destruction of her opposition. When Robinson became head of state, birth control was still illegal in Ireland, married women were barred from holding certain government jobs, and the gender wage gap was about two to one in favor of men.

President from 1990 to 1997, Robinson played a significant part in liberalizing Ireland. She also fundamentally altered relations with England, being the first Irish president to meet with a British monarch, Queen Elizabeth II. Throughout her time as president and afterward, serving as UN high commissioner for Human Rights, she achieved tremendous popularity in Ireland. In 2019 on the occasion of her seventy-fifth birthday, *Irish Central* dubbed her "the most consequential Irish woman of the 20th century."[9]

When Mary Robinson was inaugurated as president on December 3, 1990, she gave a speech in which she told a story of the Irish nation.[10] It was a story about where Ireland was coming from and where the Irish people were headed, and it situated her own leadership as embodying their journey from a restrictive and insular past to a tolerant and vibrant future.

> The Ireland I will be representing is a new Ireland, open, tolerant, inclusive. Many of you who voted for me did so without sharing all of my views. This, I believe, is a significant signal of change, a sign, however modest, that we have already passed the threshold to a new pluralist Ireland.

Like all leaders, Robinson made use of boundaries to define her group. But she did so in a radically inclusive way, casting a net much wider than just the nation-state to bring the "vast community of Irish emigrants" around the world—wherever they might be—into the identity.

She further expanded her nation's story to include an ambitious vision for the role Ireland would play on the world stage. The Berlin Wall had fallen just one year earlier and she noted that she was taking office "at a vital moment in Europe's history." Might not Ireland, with its commitment to human rights, tolerance, and inclusivity, have a critical role to play in the reshaping of Europe under her leadership?

> May I have the fortune to preside over an Ireland at a time of exciting transformation when we enter a new Europe where old wounds can be healed, a time when, in the words of Seamus Heaney, "hope and history rhyme." May it be a Presidency where I the President can sing to you, citizens of Ireland, the joyous

refrain of the fourteenth-century Irish poet as recalled by W. B. Yeats: "I am of Ireland...come dance with me in Ireland."

Robinson understood that the language that leaders use, whether spoken, written, or tweeted, is a vital tool for crafting a shared identity.

When we hear or read powerful speeches, we tend to focus on the well-turned phrase, the apt metaphor, the beautiful, even poetic rhythms. These features demark great oratory. But more subtle linguistic cues matter too, in particular the use of words that signal solidarity.

Researchers Viviane Seyranian and Michelle Bligh coded speeches from every twentieth-century American president, from Teddy Roosevelt through George W. Bush, for the use of inclusive language.[11] They were on the lookout for words and phrases that invoked collective identities as well as similarity between leader and followers.

First, though, they asked ten political scientists to determine which of the seventeen presidents had been "charismatic leaders." Charismatic leaders, as the researchers put it, "institute social change and change the status quo in some fundamental way...by presenting people with a powerful vision that inspires and motivates them." Only five presidents were deemed charismatic by these criteria: both Roosevelts, John F. Kennedy, Ronald Reagan, and Bill Clinton.

When the researchers examined the presidents' speeches, they found that these five used significantly more inclusive language than the other twelve. This was true throughout their terms in office, although the charismatic presidents were especially likely to use language invoking similarity to their followers earlier on in their tenures. It may have been most important to establish themselves as embodying the group while their presidencies were still young, much as Mary Robinson did in her inaugural address.

Research suggests that the language of identity may be a winning strategy. In 2013, researchers analyzed the campaign speeches of every winner and loser who had sought to become Australia's prime minister since 1901. Victors in these elections used collective pronouns ("we" and "us"), as opposed to individual pronouns ("I" and "me"), significantly more often than the candidates who lost.[12] On average, politicians who won these races said "we" or "us" once every 79 words in their speeches, compared to once every 136 words for the runners-up—nearly twice as frequently.

Leaders use language to crystallize this shared sense of purpose, and leaders we think of as iconic are also alive to the power of a moment to signify the social identity they hope to bring to life through their followers. Around the same time that Mary Robinson was articulating a new vision for the Irish identity, a leader on another continent and in very different circumstances harnessed the same principles of identity leadership to help lift his country out of an incredibly dark period of history.

IDENTITY SYMBOLS

As South Africa's apartheid regime began to disintegrate in the early 1990s, the country was isolated and in crisis. Sanctions imposed by other nations to protest the regime's brutal racist policies had decimated the economy. Alliances of convenience with Western countries against the Soviets had dissolved with the end of the Cold War. Political violence—protest and repression both—threatened to destabilize the nation. A descent into civil war was entirely possible.

Into this nerve-racking environment, where any false move might lead to mass violence, Nelson Mandela emerged. Mandela had spent twenty-six years in prison for his opposition to the apartheid regime, confined for stretches to a cell less than fifty square feet on the notorious Robben Island. Mandela had lost a great deal. He had missed watching his children grow up. And when his mother and eldest son died a year apart, he was not allowed to attend either of their funerals.

To Black South Africans and supporters of his party, the African

National Congress, Mandela was a heroic figure. But to many White South Africans, he was a criminal and a terrorist. They felt great unease—even fear—when Mandela was released from prison in 1990, and they felt it again in 1994 when, following the opening of free elections, Mandela was voted in as president of South Africa. What would he and the African National Congress do now that they had swept to power and were suddenly in control?

Nelson Mandela was, fortunately, not a man inclined to exact revenge on his oppressors. He was a leader who understood the power of identity symbols to not only divide people, as they had done for generations in his country, but also bring them together.

The year after Mandela's election, South Africa hosted the Rugby World Cup. During the apartheid era, South Africa had been banned from competition, so this was a symbolic event. But Mandela recognized that it could be more meaningful still. The South African team, the Springboks—then a Whites-only team—were beloved by White South Africans and widely despised by the Black population, who would often cheer for the opposing side on principle.

So when the Springboks competed for—and eventually won—the Rugby World Cup on their home turf, Mandela seized the moment. In a gesture immortalized in the film *Invictus,* he stepped out to the podium not just as president of the country but also as a fan— wearing the distinctive green Springbok cap and jersey.

To Black and White South Africans alike, Mandela's action was a simple but profound statement: We are one team and we are one country. In this moment, Mandela was able to co-opt a symbol of colonial oppression and use it to bring his country a bit closer together.

Of course, not all leaders draw the boundaries as inclusively as Mary Robinson and Nelson Mandela did. Some leaders seek to mobilize narrower coalitions, using stark "us" versus "them" distinctions to create more exclusionary social identities. Leaders may try to strengthen internal cohesion by drawing attention to intergroup competition and perceived threats from the outside. We see this dynamic, of course, in polarized political systems and authoritarian regimes. But it is nothing new and we will discuss its dangers at the end of this chapter when we talk about leadership gone bad.

As inspiring as figures like Mandela and Robinson are, there is a danger of focusing too much on stories, words, and symbols, on grand rhetorical gestures. Howard Gardner's idea of embodiment reminds us that leaders' actions matter as much as their words. The identity stories they tell, the way they use language, invoke symbols, and frame boundaries, are unlikely to rally followers to their cause if they are inconsistent with these leaders' own choices.

WORDS INTO ACTION

A cowardly leader cannot instill courage. A selfish leader will not inspire generosity. And leaders who do not invest resources or support vaunted initiatives with concrete action will ultimately fail.

More generally, effective leaders are highly attentive to creating the conditions, structures, and institutions needed to make their identity stories real. Nelson Mandela didn't just put on the green Springboks jersey and call it a day. South African leaders approached the long and arduous process of healing and unifying their country in a deep and deliberative way. Recognizing that the past doesn't remain in the past unless it is confronted, they established mechanisms like the Truth and Reconciliation Commission to grapple with the nation's horrific history of apartheid and thus help to secure a more hopeful future. Rosa Parks and her compatriots in the civil rights movement organized, organized, organized, and organized some more. In addition to being prime minister during World War II, Churchill took the title of minister of defense. From this position, he oversaw nearly every element of the war effort, from naval strategy and weapons development to food rationing and press coverage. More recently, Jacinda Ardern and her government took over every logistical element involved in keeping COVID-19 under control in New Zealand.

The principle of aligning conditions, structures, and processes with the group's identity applies equally in organizations and companies. Many companies are eager to increase diversity and create more inclusive and equitable cultures. But hosting some workshops and posting an expression of values online is not enough. To make serious headway, leaders must use the full range of the managerial tools at their disposal to make this story of "who we are becoming" concrete and put the weight of action behind the vision. Allocate adequate resources to equity initiatives, which means not just hiring a diversity, equity, and inclusion officer but providing that person with a significant budget and decision-making authority. Audit and change processes that might be introducing bias. Monitor the environment for progress toward and setbacks from these goals. Request regular updates on who is being hired and, perhaps more important, who is being retained. Look out for warning signs that members of underrepresented groups are not thriving in your organization, and do so visibly. Insist on finding and rooting out underlying and systemic contributors to these problems.

All of these are ways that leaders embody, in the day-to-day moments of doing their jobs, the identities that they are striving to create. Another way leaders exemplify and reinforce these identities is in their response when the group's sense of shared reality— perhaps its very definition—is threatened.

RESPONDING TO THREATS

Although it is rarely noted as such, one of the most iconic moments of leadership studied by social psychologists occurred in the early-morning hours of December 21, 1954, when Dorothy Martin rallied the sagging spirits of her doomsday cult. We heard their story in chapter 3.[13] This group of believers had expected to be rescued from Earth by alien spacecraft at the stroke of midnight. They were devastated when the moment came and went without an alien in sight.

But shortly thereafter Ms. Martin received an interstellar message that their little group, sitting all night long, had spread so much light that the world had been saved. Their shared reality was rescued from the brink: *We are not crazy; we are wise and good. We are heroes, even.*

Protecting and bolstering their groups' shared conceptions of themselves is something that leaders are called on to do on a regular basis. In particular, leaders respond creatively when events, internal or external, threaten the group's identity.[14]

One such threat shook American business schools in 1988 when, for the very first time, *Business Week* began to rank management programs.[15] The magazine used a scale with two key metrics: recent MBA graduates' satisfaction with their programs and the satisfaction that corporate recruiters had in those graduates. Suddenly the complex array of business-school identities—containing rich conceptions of who the institutions were and their sense of self-worth—was collapsed into a single dimension. Their value was reduced to a stark and solitary number.

Prior to this, every school could take pride in what it saw as its unique strengths. Perhaps they saw themselves as incubators of national leaders or research-intensive programs or regional powerhouses. By differentiating and highlighting what made it unique, every school could conceive of itself as among the very best. In the words of John Byrne, the man who created the rankings: "For years and years there were probably 50 business schools that claimed they were in the top 20 and probably hundreds that claimed they were in the top 40.... The *Business Week* survey eliminated the ability of some schools to claim they were in a top group."[16]

The new rankings produced dismay among business-school

247

leaders, particularly those who saw their positive beliefs about their schools reduced to an unflattering number. Organizational psychologists Kim Elsbach and Roderick Kramer took advantage of this sudden new identity threat to examine how leaders of these institutions responded.

The researchers analyzed documents, such as press releases and articles in student newspapers, and interviewed deans and public relations professionals. Said one: "It was a travesty." Said another: "I wouldn't be dean of this institution for very long if I did nothing to respond to even the *perception* that our school was slipping in its national standing."

In response, business-school leaders challenged the very notion that their organizations could legitimately be compared en masse without attention to more specific categories. As one put it, "*Business Week* is throwing the Fords and the Chevys and the Porsches in the same mix. It's not really fair. It's like judging apples and oranges, and we're not the same type of school as many others." Further, if there had to be rankings, they suggested more appropriate comparisons. Not coincidentally, these tended to be ones that cast their own schools in a positive light.

Perhaps more important, however, business-school leaders took advantage of the threat to reinforce their followers' shared conceptions of who they were. They doubled down on their internally shared realities. An administrator at the University of California, Berkeley, for example, said: "We really value our *entrepreneurial culture* around here. It's central to how we see ourselves. If the Haas [Business School] emphasis on high tech and entrepreneurship was to change, the school would lose its identity and competitive advantage." In other words: *We will not let others define us; we are not generic; we are not like everyone else, and we must maintain our distinctive identity.*

To this point, we have discussed how leaders can make use of the tools of social identity to build solidarity and animate their groups. But does it work? Not all leaders are equally inspiring to their followers, and, ultimately, it is followers' reactions that determine a leader's success. Followers evaluate leaders through the lenses of their social identities and follow these leaders, at least with enthusiasm, only if they trust them.

THE ESSENCE OF LEADERSHIP

As we have seen, one of the key consequences of shared identities is that they encourage people to trust one another. The sense that you can safely rely on someone else is especially important when the outcome, perhaps even your fate, lies in another person's hands. For this reason, people tend to be particularly concerned about the trustworthiness of their leaders, who control the futures of their teams, organizations, and nations.[17]

Trust in leaders matters beyond the trust that people who share an identity have in each other. Kurt Dirks, a scientist at Simon Fraser University, convinced the head coaches of thirty men's NCAA basketball teams to let him survey their players before the start of the conference season.[18] Three hundred and thirty players rated how much they trusted their coach, among other things.

Dirks tracked each team's performance and found that teams whose players agreed that "most members of the team trust and respect the coach" and "the coach approaches his job with professionalism and dedication" performed better. Indeed, teams' trust in their coaches at the beginning of the season predicted winning a greater proportion of games during the season and it did so even when controlling for a host of other variables in the analysis, including players' trust in each other, the overall level of talent on the team, coaches' prior records of performance, and how the team itself had performed in the past.

Something one of the players said is illuminating: "Once we developed trust in [our coach], the progress we made increased tremendously because we were no longer asking questions or were apprehensive. Instead, we were buying in and believe that if we worked our hardest, we were going to get there."[19]

In other words, trusting their leaders allows groups to capitalize on the benefits of having a leader in the first place. There is someone to set the direction and make key decisions so the rest of the team can buckle down and do their jobs. It is not a shock, therefore, that research in the workplace shows that trust in leaders is associated with a number of good things, including better job performance, more altruism, higher satisfaction and commitment, and lower turnover.

Unsurprisingly, in the NCAA basketball analysis, teams that had performed better in the past also won more games during the season under investigation. What is perhaps more surprising was that this relationship seemed, statistically speaking, to run through trust in the coach. Doing well in the past was associated with doing well in the future in part because it increased how much people trusted the leader in the present. Great leadership produces a virtuous cycle: trustworthy leaders promote success, we trust leaders who have helped us be successful, and that trust helps generate future success.

Believing that our leaders are doing good things for us, like helping us win, is one key reason we trust them. Research suggests that another important factor is how "prototypic" they are—or how much they appear to be *one of us*.[20] When people identify with a group, they perceive key characteristics of the group to be self-defining. If a core component of your group's identity involves being conscientious or competitive or curious, you will tend to see yourself that way. So, too, will you adjust your behavior to align with group norms. But of course, within any group there is variation between people in terms of how well they exemplify core-defining traits and norms.

It turns out that groups are often especially attuned to how well their leaders "fit" their social identities. Psychologists are careful to refer to this fit as *prototypicality* rather than *typicality* because the most trusted and influential leaders are not the most average of group members and they are not just trying to fit in. Instead, they are among those who best capture the *essence* of who the group members think they are, or who they want to be. Indeed, leaders often achieve this in an exaggerated fashion by being more like "one of us" than the rest of the group: a living, breathing encapsulation of the group's social identity.

A superficial version of this occurs when politicians try to secure photo ops of themselves eating down-to-earth and local cuisine—a hot dog, cheesesteak, or pizza—during election campaigns. Done well, however, the fit between leader and group is authentic. The genuine sense that our leader understands us, can speak for us, and will make choices that reflect our best interests gives followers the confidence to be led.

Unfortunately, there can be a major downside to using fit to decide who should be trusted as a leader. Too strong a focus on matching a particular prototype may limit the leadership opportunities that are afforded to people who do not appear similar to the majority or to traditional conceptions of the group. In industries historically dominated by White males, for example, women and members of underrepresented racial or ethnic groups may be perceived as less worthy of promotion or as performing less well as leaders.[21]

Research also suggests that when people feel uncertain, they tend to prefer prototypic leaders. One exception to this can occur when groups experience a crisis that causes them to think that they need a different sort of person in charge. In this situation, they might conclude that it is time for a change.[22] In moments of poor corporate performance, for example, organizations may decide to replace their male CEOs with female leaders. This sounds like it could be a good thing. But Michelle Ryan and her colleagues have found that very often, it is far from positive.[23] In many cases, those non-prototypical leaders are being set up for failure.

Their work demonstrates a "glass cliff" effect in which women and other underrepresented leaders are indeed more likely to be promoted in times of poor performance and organizational crisis. In their words, "this is not because [women] are expected to improve the situation, but because they are seen to be good people managers and can take the blame for organizational failure." As a result, female leaders are disproportionately set up to take the fall for bad situations they did not create and that they may struggle to fix, as would any leader in the same circumstances. And, of course, if they do fail, it perpetuates old stereotypes that men are better leaders than women.

To get past this, conceptions of what it means to be "one of us" need to broaden. Thankfully, groups' notions of what is "good for us" are not fixed. They can decide that bringing a diversity of experiences, backgrounds, and knowledge to leadership is important. They can decide that they want their groups to grow and evolve in their vision and membership.

Finally, in addition to trusting leaders who do good things for us and who appear to be one of us, we trust leaders who play fair. Leaders often have to make tough decisions, decisions with real consequences for the lives of their followers. They decide which basketball players to keep on the bench. They decide who gets a promotion and who does not. They may have to lay people off. They might even decide to go to war.

The concept of *procedural justice* recognizes that there is a difference between the way leaders make decisions and the actual decisions they make—and followers care a lot about both of these things.[24] Making decisions in a procedurally just way is key to securing and maintaining trust. Even when people do not like a decision, it is more palatable if it is made in a way that they see as fair. They are more willing to accept outcomes contrary to their interests, such as not getting a promotion or a job, as long as they think the process was fair.

People perceive decision-making as fair when it appears to be neutral, when the leader seems to have no ulterior motive, and when they are given courtesy and respect. The way people are treated when decisions are made sends a message about how their leaders view them and about their standing in the group. Being treated rudely and subjected to biased or arbitrary processes signals that clearly you do not matter. Being treated politely with careful and unbiased procedures shows that you are valued, even if it did not turn out the way you had hoped. Unsurprisingly, the people with the strongest social identities, the ones who are most invested in the group and their standing within it, tend to care the most about being treated fairly.

A great deal of leadership, then, involves followers' social identities, which can be harnessed to influence how they think, feel, and act. But leaders can be heavily influenced by social identities too— the social identity of their group as well as how they understand themselves as members of a category of leaders.

LEADERS' OWN IDENTITIES

Social identities shape perceptions and what people pay attention to. Identities motivate members to protect certain conceptions of their group and maintain shared realities. People can, at times, enter identity-affirming echo chambers that blind them to alternate perspectives. As deeply invested, often highly prototypic group members themselves, leaders are affected by all of these processes as well.[25] For example, a group's sense of its shared reality can influence how its leaders monitor their environments, affecting what opportunities they see as well as which threats they perceive.

In 1970, Intel became the first company to produce commercially available dynamic random-access memory (known as DRAM). This new technology was a huge improvement on the magnetic forms of memory that computers had previously used. DRAM technology launched Intel as a major player in the computing industry, and for a time DRAM was the core of its business. But by the early 1980s, Intel had come under heavy competition from Japanese tech companies, which steadily eroded Intel's share of the market. In an analysis examining how organizations respond to strategic challenges, Robert Burgelman and former Intel CEO Andrew Grove found that executives were slow to recognize and react to their changing competitive environment, and they attributed much of this slowness to social identity.[26]

"Top managers," they wrote, "usually rise through the ranks and are deeply influenced by their perception of what made the company successful. Intel's exit from the DRAM business, for instance, was delayed by the fact that top management was still holding on to Intel's identity as a memory company." It was not until Intel leaders realized that the company had become a microprocessor rather a memory company that they left the now unprofitable DRAM-manufacturing business behind.

In addition to identifying with the groups they lead, leaders may also possess a social identity of themselves as leaders—that is, as part of a category of people who influence others. They may cast this identity narrowly: self as CEO, self as vice president, self as prime minister. Or they may see it broadly: self as belonging to a band of leaders throughout history.

The ways that leaders understand this social identity—what it means to be a leader—can have a profound influence. Reflecting across his case studies of twentieth-century leaders, Howard Gardner noted an additional regularity. From an early age, many of these leaders seem to have perceived themselves as rightfully belonging to this category, as deserving a place within it. Indeed, Gardner identifies this characteristic as part of the leader identity prototype, describing what he terms the "exemplary leader," or "E.L.":

E.L. stands out in that she identifies with and feels herself to be a peer of an individual in a position of authority.... E.L. has pondered the issue involved in a specific position of leadership and believes that her own insights are at least as well motivated and perhaps more likely to be effective than those of the person currently at the helm.

At the age of sixteen, while talking about his future with a school-mate, Winston Churchill said, "This country will be subject somehow to a tremendous invasion, but I tell you, I shall be in command of the defenses of London and I shall save London and England from disaster."[27]

"Will you be a General then?" asked his friend.

"I don't know," replied Churchill. "Dreams of the future are blurred, but the main objective is clear. I repeat—London will be in danger and in the high position I shall occupy, it will fall to me to save the Capital and the Empire."

Spoken in 1891, this was an extraordinarily cocky but also astonishingly prescient vision of events that would occur nearly fifty years later. But this sense of identity, even destiny, as a leader does not produce complacency among those who go on to embody it. Rather, people who embrace a sense of self as leader may be especially motivated to situate themselves centrally within this category to which they desire to belong.

In his recent biography of Churchill, Andrew Roberts describes how Churchill laid out a strategic route for himself to acquire political power and how he worked at it from his teenage years onward.[28] While serving as a soldier in India, for example, Churchill brought with him and read cover to cover recent records of the British House of Commons. Preparing for the political career he anticipated, he went so far as to write his own speeches detailing what he would have said had he been in the House of Commons at the time. True to form, he pasted these hypothetical speeches into the records!

A person's sense of his or her identity as a leader may inspire great ambition and success. But too fixed an identity can also be a limitation and potential source of failure. In a case study of

President Lyndon Johnson, psychologist Roderick Kramer argues that Johnson's sense of what it meant to be a great president ultimately undermined his success in that position.[29]

Johnson undoubtedly wanted to excel and be, as he put it, "the greatest father the country ever had." And of all the U.S. presidents of the twentieth century, he was probably the most prepared in terms of skills and knowledge to achieve greatness. By the time he was sworn in after the assassination of John F. Kennedy, he had accumulated vast legislative and political experience, culminating in positions as Senate majority leader and vice president. And yet, Johnson stumbled badly over the Vietnam War. Vietnam was a conflict he inherited and did not want, yet he failed to prevent the war from escalating even as it detracted from his other priorities and made him less and less popular.

Kramer contends that "in Johnson's eyes presidential greatness had two cornerstones: a record of historic domestic achievement and the ability of a president to keep the nation out of harm's way.... [Thus] achieving greatness...required waging a successful war." It was this latter conception of presidential identity that locked Lyndon Johnson into increasing investment in a war that he knew to be a quagmire. "The thought of 'cutting and running,'" as Johnson once put it, "was anathema to someone who had such a keenly developed sense of what great, activist presidents need to do in moments of crisis and challenge."

THE GOOD, THE UGLY, AND THE BAD

Lyndon Johnson may have been too caught up in his concept of what it meant to be a great president, but leaders can struggle and fail for many reasons. We do not offer a comprehensive account of leaders' shortcomings, but thinking about how leaders can harness social identities highlights several ways they can go astray.

Perhaps most common, people in leadership positions may simply neglect social identity altogether, failing to capitalize on its potential to build solidarity, grow trust, and mobilize people around a common purpose. In our experience, even people who are praised as good leaders often focus much more on the individual-enhancing side of transformational leadership than the group-enhancing side. These are bosses who carefully develop and appropriately recognize their followers as individuals but fail to articulate a compelling collective vision or help the group members work well together. They tend to run their teams by maintaining strong one-to-one relationships with followers without doing much to help them see themselves as a whole, greater than the sum of its parts.

These leaders miss an opportunity. But these leaders are, of course, vastly preferable to leaders who are actively destructive of social identity and, indeed, of interpersonal relationships. One leadership style of this type has been described as "petty tyranny."[30] *Tyranny* because these people exploit their power at the expense of others, and *petty* because it's unnecessary and often over trivial things. Most of us have had the misfortune to encounter at least one person like this.

In a meta-analysis on the effects of destructive leadership in the workplace, Birgit Schyns and Jan Schilling found that employees felt negatively toward hostile and obstructive supervisors and were likely to resist following them.[31] Importantly, they also found that employees whose leaders were rated as destructive felt more negatively toward their organizations as a whole and engaged in more "counterproductive work behavior." Counterproductive work behavior is a polite way of describing actions that range from slacking off to outright fraud and theft. These findings suggest that badly behaved bosses not only poison their own relationships with followers, they damage identification with the whole group as well.

Well-intentioned leaders who do not take social identity seriously enough are the good (but not great). Tyrannical and destructive leaders are the ugly, people who are definitely not well intentioned and who are apt to create a hot mess wherever they go. But there is a third and much more dangerous species of leader: those who know how to harness social identities, who are good at building solidarity and cohesion among their followers, and who do so for corrupt, unethical, or immoral purposes. For, as we have seen, social identities can be a force for good or a force for evil. In the hands of the wrong people, powerful identity stories can lead groups badly astray.

TYRANNY AND RESISTANCE

One by one, the nine young men were rounded up. Palo Alto police officers arrested them at their homes and charged them with armed robbery and burglary. This marked the beginning of another of the most famous experiments in the history of psychology.[32]

In the summer of 1971, eighteen healthy young men responded to an advertisement calling for volunteers for a "psychological study of prison life." It paid fifteen dollars a day for one to two weeks in late August and was designed to simulate the experience of living and working in a prison. The men were randomly assigned, by the flip of a coin, to play the role of either prisoner or guard.

The charismatic young psychologist Philip Zimbardo and his research assistants built a realistic mock prison, complete with cells and shackles, in the basement of Stanford University's psychology department. Picked up by the police, a flourish designed to add realism, the prisoners were transported to this jail. They were met there by the guards, who fingerprinted them, strip-searched them, and provided them with new identities in the form of ID numbers.

According to the legend presented in most textbooks, "the guards were given no specific training on how to be guards." They were provided with dark glasses and billy clubs and let loose while the experimenters watched to see what would happen. Famously, over the next few days, the guards began to treat the prisoners with increasing disrespect and aggression. This triggered a brief uprising by the prisoners, after which the guards cracked down with escalating brutality. Misbehaving prisoners were placed in "the Hole," a four-foot-square closet the guards repurposed for solitary confinement. Others were subjected to humiliation as well as physical and sexual harassment. The guards grew more savage, the prisoners more submissive.

Things became so toxic that Zimbardo shut down the experiment after only six days.

Based on this version of events, the conclusion is obvious: People are powerfully affected, perhaps automatically, by the roles they are given. Provide someone with a uniform and dark glasses and call him or her a guard, and the brutal treatment of prisoners is almost an inevitability.

This idea—that roles have near inescapable consequences—has spread far and wide.[33] It has been taught to millions of students around the world; it has been argued in court cases, depicted in popular films, described in bestselling books, and presented to Congress. The idea that people naturally conform to their social roles and that this can cause malfeasance or cruelty is often invoked when people in positions of authority misbehave.

But this idea that roles or identities have inevitable effects on behavior should, by now, sound problematic to you. How people behave when they take on an identity is influenced by group norms and by leadership. Indeed, leaders are fundamentally involved in establishing, promoting, and enforcing particular types of norms.

Half a century after the Stanford Prison Experiment, we have new information that puts the study in an entirely different light.[34] Recently, Jay got involved in research with Stephen Reicher and Alex Haslam, analyzing the release of new tapes and documents from Stanford University's archives. It turns out that the participants in the famous study were not simply let loose without guidance. Quite the contrary. Our analysis has instead revealed the striking role that identity leadership played in how the experiment turned out.

Such leadership began shortly after the prisoners arrived. Dr. Zimbardo himself served as the prison superintendent, and his research assistants were appointed as prison wardens. When the experiment began, the superintendent gave clear instructions to his guard followers:

> You can create in the prisoners feelings of boredom, a sense of fear to some degree, you can create a notion of arbitrariness that their life is totally controlled by us.... They'll have no freedom of action, they can do nothing, say nothing we don't permit.

In the archives, we discovered and analyzed a fascinating audio recording of a conversation between an experimenter known as Warden Jaffe and one of the guard participants.[35] Despite the popular notion that the guards spontaneously became brutal toward the prisoners, this was not the case. This particular guard was reluctant to embrace his assigned role and behave as aggressively as the researchers leading the study wanted him to.

Warden Jaffe calls the guard to task: "We really want to get you active and involved because the guards have to know that every guard is going to be what we call a tough guard and so far..." The guard replies, "I'm not too tough." "Yeah," says the warden, "well, you have to try to kind of get it in you."

In their conversation (of which this exchange is just a short snippet), the warden encouraged the guard to see himself as sharing the same goals and values as the experimenters. This strategy involved situating the experiment within a broader moral and worthy purpose. He explained that the experiment was designed to provide information that would improve the correctional system out in the real world. Their research was intended, he said, to make real prisons more humane by exposing their brutality. This was a virtuous mission!

Most striking, at least to us, were the ways in which the warden employed the tools of identity leadership to encourage the reluctant guard to become more aggressive. The warden used collective pronouns fifty-seven times (once every thirty words) to try to communicate that he and the guard were in this together, on the same team. For as we have seen, this type of communal language communicates a sense of cohesion and solidarity.

The discovery of these materials dramatically changes the conclusions we draw from this famous study. Many of the guards did indeed end up behaving brutally toward the prisoners, but their behavior was by no means inevitable or automatic. They were coaxed into aggressive action by leaders who framed the study as an "us" versus "them" situation, actively intervened when their followers resisted, used the language of identity, and built norms of brutality.

The Stanford Prison Experiment is a microcosm of some of the processes involved when social identities turn ugly. Haslam and Reicher have described a progression of stages by which leaders move their groups toward evil, ultimately culminating in violence or even genocide.[36] The initial steps are common and relatively benign. Leaders foster a cohesive group identity, in part by establishing boundaries between "us" and "them." Boundaries are not inherently problematic. After all, competition between sports teams, between companies, and between nations at events like the Olympics all make boundaries highly salient.

Boundaries become perilous when leaders define outsiders as threats, convincing followers that they pose a significant, even existential, danger to the beloved group. The peril is often particularly acute when leaders' rhetoric excludes people who would otherwise be included in the group. Throughout history, all manner of minority groups, including immigrants, Jews, and sexual minorities, have been targeted in this way. It is not uncommon to see groups on a trajectory toward violence starting to refer to people they have defined as outsiders as being traitors or something less than human: parasites, rats, or cockroaches.

The final stages occur in quick succession. Leaders portray their group as uniquely virtuous. *We are the source of true goodness in the world, so much so that anything we do must inherently be good. We must defend our virtue and overcome evil at all costs.* From here, it is a short step to celebrating violence and brutality as virtues. *We are the sole source of righteousness, so if outsiders threaten our goodness or our very existence, they deserve to be suppressed, oppressed, or wiped out.* Through this distorted lens, killing is presented to followers as a moral good, even an imperative.

This is how leaders throughout history have justified cruelty and aggression. The actions and language of leaders matter enormously and large-scale brutality never occurs in a vacuum.

In his book *The Anatomy of Fascism,* historian Robert Paxton described the "mobilizing passions" that produce and sustain fascist movements.[37] Among these he includes "the belief that one's group is a victim, a sentiment that justifies any action without legal or moral limits against its enemies, both internal and external.... The need for closer integration of a purer community by consent if possible or by exclusionary violence if necessary.... The superiority of the leader's instincts over abstract and universal reason."

Groups do not get here without identity leadership, reminding us that social identities can be a powerful tool for good or for evil. Yet no leader's story goes uncontested and no story is so strong that it cannot be resisted. We have focused most of this chapter on leaders whose lives and stories embodied an inclusive vision for their groups. But many of them were, of course, opposed by other potential leaders with different and sometimes more exclusionary visions.

As we said earlier, leadership can be understood, in many ways, as a battle of stories. It is incumbent on us, as followers and sometimes leaders ourselves, to decide which side of these battles we are on. We get to decide which identity stories we want to embrace, which stories about where we are coming from, where we are going, and what we must fear, struggle against, and dream of we want to live out.

CHAPTER 10

THE FUTURE OF IDENTITY

In the late 1960s, in honor of its fiftieth anniversary, the American Institute of Planners commissioned a series of papers from eminent scholars and policy makers.[1] They were asked to cast their eyes forward and write about what they saw coming over the next fifty years. Now, just over half a century later, it is fascinating to revisit what these big thinkers expected might happen. Their papers are generally a useful reminder of Mark Twain's caution that "prediction is difficult, particularly when it involves the future."

One paper was devoted to problems that might arise in the next several decades due to technological advances.[2] Some of their fears were products of the Cold War, reflecting concerns about nuclear technology and the development of some sort of "Doomsday Machine." Other forecasts seem odd, even quaint, in retrospect: worries about shock waves from supersonic jets and the dangers of million-ton tanker ships or even million-ton planes!

However, the thinkers were attentive to possibilities that have become substantive problems. They warned about growing global inequality and threats to democracy. The potential for global climate change, which they called "radical ecological changes on a planetary scale," was relegated to a miscellaneous category of "Bizarre Issues." But even here, they were prescient about the huge climate challenges we would come to face, writing that "long-term damage should be discernible in time to change what is going wrong, but it is often difficult for people to act effectively on large-scale, long-term problems, since they tend to be 'everyone's problem' and therefore, for lack of jurisdiction, no one's."

At the risk of proving Mark Twain right once again, we will offer some concluding thoughts about the future of identity. Although we know better than to try to predict the future, we will talk about the role that social identities will likely play in some of the biggest issues currently facing humanity. We will discuss economic inequality and climate change and conclude with a few thoughts about democracy.

TACKLING INEQUALITY

In 2016, the average CEO at one of America's top 350 companies took home 224 times more money than the corporation's average employee. This astonishing disparity is symbolic of growing inequalities in income and, even more, in wealth (the assets that people hold) around the world. While absolute global poverty has declined, levels of economic inequality have increased in many countries over the past several decades. By one estimate, half of the world's population possessed less than 1 percent of the world's wealth in 2018, while the richest 10 percent controlled 85 percent of it.

A recent UN report[3] concluded that 71 percent of people live in countries where inequality has increased since 1990. At the top of this list are some of the world's wealthiest nations, including the United States and the United Kingdom, where extraordinary opulence exists near but often conveniently segregated from grinding poverty and economic insecurity.

Numerous studies indicate that economic inequality is bad for individuals and bad for societies. Countries with greater inequality tend to have more violent crime, higher infant mortality, more mental illness, and lower life expectancy. The same sorts of relationships hold if you compare American states; for instance, rich but unequal California has worse outcomes on these metrics than poorer but more equal Iowa. In fact, this comparison makes a key point: It seems that inequality rather than poverty is often more powerfully associated with negative outcomes at the societal level. Societies do worse when the incomes and assets of the rich are wildly divergent from those of the poor and, increasingly, the middle class.[4]

Vast inequalities also have the potential to affect our identities. Our identities, in turn, affect our ability to grapple with and reduce economic inequality. Regarding the former, for example, while a CEO taking home millions of dollars in salary, stock options, and bonuses has reason to be pleased with life, as a leader that CEO should be concerned. Leaders, as we have seen, are able to unify and motivate their followers to the degree that they are seen as "one of us."

Can someone making 224 times what most people earn authentically be "one of us"?

Two recent studies suggest that the answer is no. In the first experiment, participants were presented with information about one of two CEOs.[5] Both were called Ruben Martin and they were the same in every way but one: whether Ruben was or was not among the nation's highest-paid chief executives. In a second study, workers reported the pay of the CEOs leading the companies they worked for. In both cases, people felt less identified with more highly paid CEOs and had less of a sense that they were good leaders. People evaluating highly paid leaders were less likely to agree that they "act as champions" or "create a sense of cohesion" than people assessing less well-remunerated executives—even if those leaders were identical in every other respect. Inequalities, in this case within organizations, can be divisive, potentially reducing leaders' abilities to build solidarity and common purpose.

At a societal level, we should care about how inequality affects people's identities at the bottom of the economic hierarchy. As we have seen, humans are status-striving animals, seeking to possess positively regarded and respected identities. To the degree that being in a low socioeconomic bracket signals lower status in society, identifying oneself as such might have negative consequences for well-being. Indeed, in a recent analysis, psychologists at Australia's University of Newcastle found that lower socioeconomic status was associated with more anxiety and less life satisfaction.[6] But this pattern was only observed for people who said that their social class was an important part of their identity and that it was something they thought about often.

More broadly, social commentators have long speculated that poorer people's feelings of "relative deprivation," the sense that they are receiving less than others, produce grievances that can result in antisocial attitudes and behaviors. Poorer people, for example, are often assumed to hold more negative attitudes toward minority groups and immigrants. They are also assumed to make up the dominant supporters of populist or authoritarian political movements, allegiances ostensibly driven by their economic frustration.

But it turns out that these stereotypes do not hold up to close scrutiny. In a recent book examining a broad array of evidence, social psychologists Frank Mols and Jolanda Jetten conclude that while relative deprivation can sometimes produce anti-immigrant attitudes or attraction to authoritarian leaders, "relative gratification" can do the same thing.[7] Research has found, for example, that people whose life circumstances are either declining *or* improving both report greater support for using violent tactics to secure political power. Mols and Jetten argue that these surprising reactions among people who are well off can be motivated by a desire to justify and protect their advantages, for instance by denigrating minority and marginalized groups as less deserving.

If inequality is producing widespread societal dissatisfaction and a sense that the economic hierarchy is unsustainable, attitudes and behaviors among the wealthy can be driven by fears of losing status and privilege. This is indeed a type of economic anxiety, but one that comes from a place of precarious privilege rather than poverty. It is hard not to see some of the reactionary responses to Black Lives Matter and other movements pushing for greater equality, racial and otherwise, as driven by fear of losing status.

Thinking about social movements raises the question of when economically disadvantaged people might organize for change to redress and reverse the rising inequalities of recent decades.[8] As we have seen (particularly in chapter 7), people are more likely to form a sense of collective identity around something like their socio-economic class when they perceive that being part of a particular category affects their opportunities and outcomes in life.

Societies differ in how salient social class is as a category. The United Kingdom, for example, has an old class hierarchy. In contrast, the United States possesses something of a myth of being a classless society. The American dream is one in which any child, no matter how humble his or her roots, could grow up to become a president, a CEO, a celebrity, or any other type of success. These dreams are reinforced by strong meritocratic narratives, which emphasize the role of individual pluck and luck in life. When we believe that our financial fates are largely within our control, we are less likely to rally with people of similar circumstances around a common class or economic identity, opting instead to try to do better on our own.

Of course, people do not have to rally around an entire social class in order to push for changes that would improve their economic situations. Unions, for example, organize around the interests of workers in specific industries, like steelworkers, teachers, and postal workers. But unionization rates have plummeted in the United States over the past few decades as inequality has risen. Looking to the future, we do not yet know how the rise of the so-called gig economy will affect workers' abilities to protect their rights and push for change. We suspect it will hinge, at least in part, on whether they see themselves as sharing a common fate.

Despite its new name, this type of contract work is not in any sense new, but it does appear to be on the rise due to modern technology. The development of apps that match workers with short-term jobs (delivering groceries or providing taxi services, for example) has allowed the gig economy to flourish. Because gig workers are essentially independent contractors, they typically do not receive benefits or health insurance, and it is not clear if they will be able to organize to pursue better arrangements.[9] Traditional taxi drivers banded together and formed unions. Will ride-share drivers find sufficient solidarity to fight for their collective benefits?

For groups to push for change, they need to believe that change is possible. Looking to the future, we see two things in particular that are likely to shift perceptions toward the feeling that economic change is possible, essential, and inevitable. The first of these is the COVID-19 pandemic, which, in addition to being a public health and medical catastrophe, has thrown the world economy into crisis, the depth of which is still unclear. The pandemic has deepened existing inequalities and exposed them as illegitimate. It has also created a sense of possibility—that the future will not be like the past and that this is a moment to be seized. As novelist Arundhati Roy put it, the pandemic "is a portal, a gateway between one world and the next."[10]

The second thing that probably makes fundamental economic change inevitable is climate change—the effects of which will, by most accounts, dwarf those of the pandemic.

GRAPPLING WITH CLIMATE CHANGE

On winter days, people who know where we grew up almost always say the same thing: "This must be nothing for you, you are from

Canada!" They might add "Eh?" if they're particularly sardonic. The sad truth is that after more than a decade living in the United States, we have softened, and a cold day in New York is a cold day in New York. But another reality is that winters are not quite the same as they used to be back home either. The coldest days usually are not as frigid, and the snowdrifts are not as deep as they were when we were kids. The hill where Dom learned to ski can no longer count on enough snow to open all of the slopes or even stay open all winter.

The earth has a fever and it is getting worse. The average global temperature has risen somewhere between 0.8 and 1.2 degrees Celsius since the start of the industrial revolution, and there is now near unanimous consensus among scientists that a significant proportion of this is due to human activity.[11] Despite widespread evidence for human-caused climate change, however, many people remain skeptical about its existence or importance. Indeed, even as scientific evidence accumulated during the early part of this century, the proportion of Americans who reported believing that the seriousness of climate change is exaggerated increased from 31 percent in 1998 to 48 percent in 2010, although that trend has since reversed (35 percent said it was exaggerated in 2019).[12]

Some research suggests that people who have experienced extreme weather are more likely to believe in climate change, but the effect does not seem to be terribly robust. When it comes to climate skepticism, it is not clear how much personal experiences matter. One factor that does seem to matter a great deal—at least in some places—is political identity. Conservatives in the United States, the United Kingdom, Australia, and a number of other industrialized countries are far less likely than liberals to believe that human-created climate change is a real thing.[13]

But this is not true everywhere. In an analysis examining climate beliefs in twenty-five different countries, Australian psychologist Matthew Hornsey and his colleagues found that political identity was

THE POWER OF US

not a significant factor in about three-quarters of them.[14] Political identity tended to matter more in countries with higher carbon emissions. In other words, it is in countries where the economy relies more on the consumption of fossil fuels and where, as a result, reducing the carbon footprint would have more drastic effects on day-to-day life that conservatives are less likely to believe the climate is a problem.

Of course, we should not be so naive as to think this is purely a psychological phenomenon. As the researchers put it: "One way of reading these data is that the greater the vested interests, the more likely there will be organized, funded campaigns of misinformation designed to spread the message that the 'science is not in' on climate change."[15] But these misinformation campaigns need a receptive audience, and our research suggests that partisan identity provides the lens that allows many people to accept (or reject) these claims.[16]

The 1960s planners who tried to forecast the events of the next fifty years were exactly right about the tremendous difficulty humans have tackling long-term and widespread issues like climate change. Many scientists now say that to prevent truly catastrophic damage that could ultimately render the Earth largely uninhabitable to humans, we must keep the post-industrialization rise in temperature to less than 1.5 degrees Celsius.[17]

Any hope of achieving this goal requires massive political coordination within and among nations, and it is not in the least bit clear that the identities people usually bring to political action are equipped to effectively handle these challenges. Certainly, as we have seen, partisan left-versus-right political identities are often unhelpful and destructive. But national identities, the identities with which we often confront the world stage, are also often too parochial to deal optimally with collective problems on a global scale.

It is in every nation's long-term interest to prevent catastrophic climate collapse but in no nation's immediate interest to make the hard but necessary economic, social, and political sacrifices unless everyone else does so as well. International agreements like the Paris Accords are intended to resolve these sorts of dilemmas. But, as was demonstrated by the (temporary) withdrawal of the United States—the world's second-largest emitter of carbon dioxide—from this pact in 2017, voluntary arrangements are entirely subject to the goodwill of the players and, therefore, to the vagaries of their domestic politics.

People cooperate and coordinate with one another much more readily when they see themselves as sharing an identity. The identities we activate and act upon are often those that differentiate us from others, whether they be based on boundaries of occupation, religion, race, gender, or nation. But, as we have seen, people are also drawn together by common fate, when they recognize that they share the same set of circumstances and are ultimately subject to the same destiny. Nearly eight billion people currently share this rather fragile rock circling the sun, and although the effects of climate change do not affect all communities equally, we all very much have a shared interest in saving it.

Can we capitalize on this? Can we look beyond our parochial identities? Could humans' recognition of their shared identity as residents of Earth help save the world?

Perhaps no one has experienced a truly global sense of identity more profoundly than the astronauts who have seen the Earth from space. Frank Borman, James Lovell, and William Anders spent Christmas Eve of 1968 aboard the Apollo 8 spacecraft. Just months before the first lunar landing, their mission was a practice run at orbiting the moon. As their craft circled the moon, they were mesmerized by the view of its rugged, pockmarked, almost alien surface. Then suddenly Frank Borman exclaimed, "Oh my God, look at that picture over there! There's the Earth coming up. Wow, is that pretty! You got a color film, Jim? Hand me a roll of color, quick, would you?"

The astronauts snapped a series of photos showing the Earth slowly rising over the moon's horizon. They were the first humans ever to witness an Earthrise, and when they splashed down, they brought back with them what has been called "the most influential environmental photograph ever taken."

In the half a century since, hundreds of people from thirty-eight countries have traveled to space. NASA interviewed a collection of astronauts and found that many of them had undergone "truly transformative experiences involving senses of wonder and awe, unity with nature, transcendence and universal brotherhood."[18] Although feelings of awe and transcendence are fleeting, researchers discovered that the astronauts had undergone longer-term changes in identity. They felt a deeper sense of connection with humanity as a whole. After they had seen the Earth from space, the significance of national boundaries waned and the conflicts that divide people on the ground seemed less important. As one astronaut put it, "When you go around the Earth in an hour and a half, you begin to recognize that your identity is with that whole thing."

There is no way to send everyone into space. This is perhaps unfortunate because some of our most pressing issues—not only climate change, but also pandemics, terrorism, and the potential for nuclear war—might be more easily solved if we could expand our moral circles to include much larger swaths of humanity. Indeed, research suggests that you do not have to be an astronaut to experience a sense of common human or global identity and that when people possess this highly inclusive sense of self, it is associated with more support for international cooperation and environmental protection.[19]

It seems to us, however, that these deep feelings of connection to humanity as a whole are generally too rare or too fleeting to sustain long-term and truly difficult change. For that, we will need global leadership to build a genuinely universal identity among enough of the world's peoples to overcome more parochial and narrow interests. Do humans have the psychological capacity to experience this vast an identity? Yes, we think so. But whether we will find a way to create it in time is a different story.

A WORD ABOUT DEMOCRACY

On January 6, 2021, a violent mob, egged on by the then president of the United States, attacked a joint session of Congress in an attempt to overturn the results of the presidential election. Although they were ultimately repulsed, this breach of the U.S. Capitol struck at the heart of democracy, a violent attempt to thwart the right of the people to remove their leaders and replace them with different ones.

American democracy did not die on that day, but as twenty thousand troops from the National Guard locked down Washington, DC, for the inauguration of President Biden two weeks later, it was hard to call it a peaceful transition of power. Or to believe that democracy is healthy and thriving.

Much of the past fifty years actually proved to be a golden age for democracy. While about forty countries were democracies in the late 1960s, the number grew to well over one hundred by the end of the twentieth century. In 2011, a wave of protests that came to be known as the Arab Spring roiled authoritarian regimes in the Middle East and looked like it might portend a new wave of democratization. But that has largely fizzled, and some scholars fear we may now be in a period of democratic backsliding in which countries worldwide—like Turkey, Brazil, Hungary, India, and the Philippines, among others—are moving toward less rather than more democratic participation and accountability.[20]

The big challenges we have featured in this chapter—inequality and climate change—pose dangers for democracy. As we saw, the instabilities often inherent in inequality can attract people to

273

authoritarian leadership and harden attitudes toward groups like immigrants and other marginalized communities. Meanwhile, the challenges associated with global warming, including how to cope with extreme weather, as well as likely increases in disease and the migration of populations, may also increase the appeal of strong and less democratically oriented leaders.

These trends might be amplified by technology. A recent study found that citizens' faith in their governments tends to decline when the internet arrives. In Europe, the expansion of internet access was linked to increases in votes for antiestablishment populist parties.[21]

The forecasters writing for the American Institute of Planners had a similar worry. "The world is becoming so complex and changing so rapidly and dangerously..." they wrote, "that we may be tempted to sacrifice (or may not be able to afford) democratic political processes. It is important to recall that tyrants or Caesars have frequently come to power as a result of an overwhelming desire from the mass of people for firm leadership."[22]

Certain ways of overturning democracy seem to be less popular than they used to be.[23] The number of military coups, for example, has declined over time. But while less dramatic, eroding democracy by weakening checks on executive power or by manipulating electoral processes (making it harder for certain groups to vote with restrictive rules or outright intimidation, for example) may be on the rise.

Political scientists David Waldner and Ellen Lust note that democratic backsliding occurs when "major political actors are no longer satisfied playing strictly by the rules, losing gracefully, and competing again in the next round." They go on to warn that "whether they can be constrained or whether they can continue unimpeded until democracy exists in name only depends on balances of power."[24]

Their description highlights two important questions. What motivates some political actors to want to subvert democratic rules? And how effectively can their efforts to do so be counterbalanced by other players in the political system? We suspect that identity dynamics are an important part of the story.

Political parties and their supporters may, for example, be more tempted to undermine fair and transparent electoral processes when they perceive their rivals not simply as people with different policy preferences but as dangerous or deranged—a problem that can be amplified by polarization.[25] They may start to equate the national interest with their party's interests, coming to believe that the best way of protecting the nation is by retaining power at all costs. After all, to put your country ahead of your party requires that you understand their two interests are not always one and the same—that the nation has an interest in maintaining democracy even when your own side loses an election or two.

Voters do not arrive at these perceptions spontaneously, of course. Political elites, including politicians and elements of the media, regularly exploit identity dynamics to rally followers around exclusionary identities, increasing popular support for policies that, ironically, reduce the voice of the people. And extensive polarization makes it easier to spread misinformation, conspiracy theories, and propaganda about political opponents.

Conversely, how well democratic backsliding can be resisted by counterbalancing forces is likely to be a matter of how well they can rally a multiplicity of people with diverging interests and goals around a common purpose. Can they forge a common identity in the name of democratic freedom? Can they build institutions that promote the public good, encourage cooperation, and mitigate the appeal of authoritarianism?

WHO DO WE WANT TO BE?

The future, for better or worse, will be what we make of it. It is ultimately up to people like you, the reader, to decide how you want to engage with issues like inequality, climate change, democracy, and other social problems. We believe that understanding the dynamics of social identity is essential not only to making sense of these issues but to finding solutions.

Our social identities can make us receptive to misinformation and cause us to engage in discrimination and hoard resources for our own groups. But they can also motivate us to engage in self-sacrifice, forge solidarity with others, and generate new norms for collective action. It will, of course, take leaders who understand and embrace these dynamics to mobilize people to address these—and countless other—difficult issues. It is our hope that readers like yourself will harness identity for good.

Throughout this book, we have advanced a set of identity principles. Groups are central to who we are. The most important groups in our lives and thus our most central social identities are often quite stable. And yet we also have a readiness for solidarity, which allows us to find common cause when circumstances conspire to create emergent identities. Different identities become salient to us at different times—and when a particular social identity is active, it can have profound effects. We experience the world through the lens of that identity, embrace its shared reality, and find joy in its symbols and traditions. We will sacrifice, even fight, to protect its interests. These shifts in our perceptions, beliefs, feelings, and actions often align us with the norms of the group. And when we lead and others follow, it is often by inspiring a shared sense of "who we are."

Despite their power to shape our thoughts and behaviors, our identities are also the site of our agency. Whether by rejecting or embracing a particular conception of ourselves, by challenging our groups to be better, or by organizing in solidarity to change the world, we take control of who we want to be.

ACKNOWLEDGMENTS

We owe enormous gratitude to our communities and the amazing people in them who have contributed so deeply to our identities as scientists, teachers, citizens, and human beings.

We thank our academic mentors William Cunningham, Alison Chasteen, Marilynn Brewer, Julian Thayer, and Ken Dion. You taught us just about everything we know about human psychology—and equipped us with the tools to find out more!

We thank the University of Toronto Psychology Department for assigning us as graduate students to the same small sub-basement office. Our shared experience in its musty confines helped us form an unbreakable alliance.

We especially want to acknowledge our students and the members of our labs whose questions, ideas, and energy are endlessly inspiring. Most of the work we present in this book would never have happened without you! For Dom, particular appreciation goes to Natasha Thalla, Nick Ungson, Shiang-Yi Lin, Justin Aoki, and Matthew Kugler. For Jay, particular appreciation goes to Jenny Xiao, Ana Gantman, Hannah Nam, Leor Hackel, Daniel Yudkin, Julian Wills, Billy Brady, Diego Reinero, Anni Sternisko, Elizabeth Harris and Claire Robertson, Peter Mende-Siedlecki, Oriel FeldmanHall, Andrea Periera, Philip Parnamets, Kim Doell, and Victoria Spring.

We thank our mentors, colleagues, collaborators, and friends at New York University, Lehigh University, and far beyond. Too many to list in full, you are what makes our jobs so fun and so interesting.

Acknowledgments

Thanks to Michael Wohl, Christopher Miners, and Amanda Kesek for ensuring our sanity during the many challenges of graduate school and life after.

Thanks to our outstanding agent, Jim Levine. Thanks to Marisa Vigilante, our patient and wise editor, whose help and insight produced this book. Huge appreciation also to everyone who provided advice or read bits of the book along the way, including Khalil Smith, Annie Duke, Josh Aronson, Adam Galinsky, and Sarah Grevy Gottfredsen.

Most important of all, we are eternally grateful to our patient and loving families—to Jenny, Julia, Toby, Charles, and Alison, for Dominic, and to Tessa, Jack, Annie, Matty, Brenda, and Colin, for Jay.

NOTES

CHAPTER 1: THE POWER OF US

1   Barbara Smit, *Pitch Invasion* (Harmondsworth, UK: Penguin, 2007).
2   Allan Hall, "Adidas and Puma Bury the Hatchet After 60 Years of Brothers' Feud After Football Match," *Telegraph,* September 22, 2009, https://www.telegraph.co.uk/news/worldnews/europe/germany/6216728/Adidas-and-Puma-bury-the-hatchet-after-60-years-of-brothers-feud-after-football-match.html.
3   Henri Tajfel, "Experiments in Intergroup Discrimination," *Scientific American* 223, no. 5 (1970): 96–103.
4   Henri Tajfel, "Social Identity and Intergroup Behaviour," *Social Science Information* 13, no. 2 (April 1, 1974): 65–93, https://doi.org/10.1177/053901847401300204.
5   Amélie Mummendey and Sabine Otten, "Positive-Negative Asymmetry in Social Discrimination," *European Review of Social Psychology* 9, no. 1 (1998): 107–43.
6   Jay J. Van Bavel and William A. Cunningham, "Self-Categorization with a Novel Mixed-Race Group Moderates Automatic Social and Racial Biases," *Personality and Social Psychology Bulletin* 35, no. 3 (2009): 321–35.
7   David De Cremer and Mark Van Vugt, "Social Identification Effects in Social Dilemmas: A Transformation of Motives," *European Journal of Social Psychology* 29, no. 7 (1999): 871–93, https://doi.org/10.1002/(SICI)1099-0992(199911)29:7<871::AID-EJSP962>3.0.CO;2-I.
8   Marilynn B. Brewer and Sonia Roccas, "Individual Values, Social Identity, and Optimal Distinctiveness," in *Individual Self, Relational Self, Collective Self,* ed. Constantine Sedikides and Marilynn B. Brewer (New York: Psychology Press, 2001), 219–37.
9   Lucy Maud Montgomery, *The Annotated Anne of Green Gables* (New York: Oxford University Press, 1997).
10 Jolanda Jetten, Tom Postmes, and Brendan J. McAuliffe, "'We're All Individuals': Group Norms of Individualism and Collectivism, Levels of Identification and Identity Threat," *European Journal of Social Psychology* 32, no. 2 (2002): 189–207, https://doi.org/10.1002/ejsp.65.
11 Hazel Rose Markus and Alana Conner, *Clash!: How to Thrive in a Multicultural World* (New York: Penguin, 2013).

12   Jeffrey Jones, "U.S. Clergy, Bankers See New Lows in Honesty/Ethics Ratings," Gallup.com, December 9, 2009, https://news.gallup.com/poll/124 628/Clergy-Bankers-New-Lows-Honesty-Ethics-Ratings.aspx.

13   Alain Cohn, Ernst Fehr, and Michel André Maréchal, "Business Culture and Dishonesty in the Banking Industry," *Nature* 516, no. 7529 (December 4, 2014): 86–89, https://doi.org/10.1038/nature13977.

14   Zoe Rahwan, Erez Yoeli, and Barbara Fasolo, "Heterogeneity in Banker Culture and Its Influence on Dishonesty," *Nature* 575, no. 7782 (November 2019): 345–49, https://doi.org/10.1038/s41586-019-1741-y.

15   Alain Cohn, Ernst Fehr, and Michel André Maréchal, "Selective Participation May Undermine Replication Attempts," *Nature* 575, no. 7782 (November 2019): E1–E2, https://doi.org/10.1038/s41586-019-1729-7.

CHAPTER 2: THE LENS OF IDENTITY

1   Albert H. Hastorf and Hadley Cantril, "They Saw a Game; a Case Study," *Journal of Abnormal and Social Psychology* 49, no. 1 (1954): 129–34, https://doi.org/10 .1037/h0057880.

2   Nima Mesgarani and Edward F. Chang, "Selective Cortical Representation of Attended Speaker in Multi-Talker Speech Perception," *Nature* 485, no. 7397 (May 2012): 233–36, https://doi.org/10.1038/nature11020.

3   Y. Jenny Xiao, Géraldine Coppin, and Jay J. Van Bavel, "Perceiving the World Through Group-Colored Glasses: A Perceptual Model of Intergroup Relations," *Psychological Inquiry* 27, no. 4 (October 1, 2016): 255–74, https://doi .org/10.1080/1047840X.2016.1199221.

4   Joan Y. Chiao et al., "Priming Race in Biracial Observers Affects Visual Search for Black and White Faces," *Psychological Science* 17 (May 2006): 387–92, https://doi.org/10.1111/j.1467-9280.2006.01717.x.

5   Leor M. Hackel et al., "From Groups to Grits: Social Identity Shapes Evaluations of Food Pleasantness," *Journal of Experimental Social Psychology* 74 (January 1, 2018): 270–80, https://doi.org/10.1016/j.jesp.2017.09.007.

6   Ibid.

7   Kristin Shutts et al., "Social Information Guides Infants' Selection of Foods," *Journal of Cognition and Development* 10, nos. 1–2 (2009): 1–17.

8   Géraldine Coppin et al., "Swiss Identity Smells like Chocolate: Social Identity Shapes Olfactory Judgments," *Scientific Reports* 6, no. 1 (October 11, 2016): 34979, https://doi.org/10.1038/srep34979.

9   Stephen D. Reicher et al., "Core Disgust Is Attenuated by Ingroup Relations," *Proceedings of the National Academy of Sciences* 113, no. 10 (March 8, 2016): 2631–35, https://doi.org/10.1073/pnas.1517027113.

10   Ibid.

11   Y. Jenny Xiao and Jay J. Van Bavel, "See Your Friends Close and Your Enemies Closer: Social Identity and Identity Threat Shape the Representation of Physical Distance," *Personality and Social Psychology Bulletin* 38, no. 7 (July 1, 2012): 959–72, https://doi.org/10.1177/0146167212442228.

12   Y. Jenny Xiao, Michael J. A. Wohl, and Jay J. Van Bavel, "Proximity Under Threat: The Role of Physical Distance in Intergroup Relations," *PLOS ONE*

11, no. 7 (July 28, 2016): e0159792, https://doi.org/10.1371/journal.pone
.0159792.

13   "Trump Leads 'Build That Wall' Chant in California," NBC News, May 25,
2016, https://www.nbcnews.com/video/trump-leads-build-that-wall-chant
-in-california-692809283877.

14   Xiao and Van Bavel, "See Your Friends Close and Your Enemies Closer."

15   Xiao, Wohl, and Van Bavel, "Proximity Under Threat."

16   Conor Friedersdorf, "The Killing of Kajieme Powell and How It Divides
Americans," *Atlantic*, August 21, 2014, https://www.theatlantic.com/national
/archive/2014/08/the-killing-of-kajieme-powell/378899/.

17   David Yokum, Anita Ravishankar, and Alexander Coppock, "A Randomized
Control Trial Evaluating the Effects of Police Body-Worn Cameras," *Proceedings of the National Academy of Sciences* 116, no. 21 (2019): 10329–32.

18   Timothy Williams et al., "Police Body Cameras: What Do You See?," *New York Times*, April 1, 2016, https://www.nytimes.com/interactive/2016/04
/01/us/police-bodycam-video.html.

19   Yael Granot et al., "Justice Is Not Blind: Visual Attention Exaggerates Effects
of Group Identification on Legal Punishment," *Journal of Experimental Psychology: General* 143, no. 6 (2014): 2196–208, https://doi.org/10.1037
/a0037893.

20   Emma Pierson et al., "A Large-Scale Analysis of Racial Disparities in Police
Stops Across the United States," *Nature Human Behaviour* 4, no. 7 (July 2020):
736–45, https://doi.org/10.1038/s41562-020-0858-1.

21   Bocar A. Ba et al., "The Role of Officer Race and Gender in Police-Civilian
Interactions in Chicago," *Science* 371, no. 6530 (February 12, 2021): 696–702,
https://doi.org/10.1126/science.abd8694.

22   Mahzarin R. Banaji and Anthony G. Greenwald, *Blindspot: Hidden Biases of Good People* (New York: Bantam, 2016).

CHAPTER 3: SHARING REALITY

1   Leon Festinger, Henry Riecken, and Stanley Schachter, *When Prophecy Fails*
(New York: Harper and Row, 1964).

2   Solomon E. Asch, "Studies of Independence and Conformity: I. A Minority
of One Against a Unanimous Majority," *Psychological Monographs: General and Applied* 70, no. 9 (1956): 1–70; Solomon E. Asch, "Opinions and Social Pressure," *Scientific American* 193, no. 5 (1955): 31–35.

3   Robert S. Baron, Joseph A. Vandello, and Bethany Brunsman, "The Forgotten Variable in Conformity Research: Impact of Task Importance on Social
Influence," *Journal of Personality and Social Psychology* 71, no. 5 (1996): 915–27,
https://doi.org/10.1037/0022-3514.71.5.915.

4   Joachim I. Krueger and Adam L. Massey, "A Rational Reconstruction of Misbehavior," *Social Cognition* 27, no. 5 (2009): 786–812, https://doi.org/10
.1521/soco.2009.27.5.786.

5   Sushil Bikhchandani, David Hirshleifer, and Ivo Welch, "A Theory of Fads,
Fashion, Custom, and Cultural Change as Informational Cascades," *Journal of Political Economy* 100, no. 5 (1992): 992–1026.

6   Dominic Abrams et al., "Knowing What to Think by Knowing Who You Are: Self-Categorization and the Nature of Norm Formation, Conformity and Group Polarization," *British Journal of Social Psychology* 29, no. 2 (1990): 97–119; Dominic J. Packer, Nick D. Ungson, and Jessecae K. Marsh, "Conformity and Reactions to Deviance in the Time of COVID-19," *Group Processes and Intergroup Relations* 24, no. 2 (2021): 311–17.

7   Jonah Berger and Chip Heath, "Who Drives Divergence? Identity Signaling, Outgroup Dissimilarity, and the Abandonment of Cultural Tastes," *Journal of Personality and Social Psychology* 95, no. 3 (September 2008): 593–607, https://doi.org/10.1037/0022-3514.95.3.593.

8   Philip Fernbach and Steven Sloman, "Why We Believe Obvious Untruths," *New York Times,* March 3, 2017, https://www.nytimes.com/2017/03/03/opinion/sunday/why-we-believe-obvious-untruths.html.

9   Jamie L. Vernon, "On the Shoulders of Giants," *American Scientist,* June 19, 2017, https://www.americanscientist.org/article/on-the-shoulders-of-giants.

10   Kenneth Warren, *Bethlehem Steel: Builder and Arsenal of America* (Pittsburgh: University of Pittsburgh Press, 2010).

11   Carol J. Loomis, Patricia Neering, and Christopher Tkaczyk, "The Sinking of Bethlehem Steel," *Fortune,* April 5, 2004, https://money.cnn.com/magazines/fortune/fortune_archive/2004/04/05/366339/index.htm.

12   Bill Keller, "Enron for Dummies," *New York Times,* January 26, 2002, https://www.nytimes.com/2002/01/26/opinion/enron-for-dummies.html; "Understanding Enron," *New York Times,* January 14, 2002, https://www.nytimes.com/2002/01/14/business/understanding-enron.html.

13   Dennis Tourish and Naheed Vatcha, "Charismatic Leadership and Corporate Cultism at Enron: The Elimination of Dissent, the Promotion of Conformity and Organizational Collapse," *Leadership* 1 (November 1, 2005): 455–80, https://doi.org/10.1177/1742715005057671.

14   Ibid.

15   Peter C. Fusaro and Ross M. Miller, *What Went Wrong at Enron: Everyone's Guide to the Largest Bankruptcy in U.S. History* (Hoboken, NJ: John Wiley and Sons, 2002).

16   Ned Augenblick et al., "The Economics of Faith: Using an Apocalyptic Prophecy to Elicit Religious Beliefs in the Field," National Bureau of Economic Research, December 21, 2012, https://doi.org/10.3386/w18641.

17   Festinger, Riecken, and Schachter, *When Prophecy Fails.*

18   Anni Sternisko, Aleksandra Cichocka, and Jay J. Van Bavel, "The Dark Side of Social Movements: Social Identity, Non-Conformity, and the Lure of Conspiracy Theories," *Current Opinion in Psychology* 35 (2020): 1–6.

19   Paul 't Hart, "Irving L. Janis' Victims of Groupthink," *Political Psychology* 12, no. 2 (1991): 247–78, https://doi.org/10.2307/3791464.

20   Keith E. Stanovich, Richard F. West, and Maggie E. Toplak, "Myside Bias, Rational Thinking, and Intelligence," *Current Directions in Psychological Science* 22, no. 4 (2013): 259–64.

21   Roderick M. Kramer, "Revisiting the Bay of Pigs and Vietnam Decisions 25 Years Later: How Well Has the Groupthink Hypothesis Stood the Test of Time?," *Organizational Behavior and Human Decision Processes* 73, nos. 2–3 (February 1998): 236–71, https://doi.org/10.1006/obhd.1998.2762.

22 Jonathan Haidt, "New Study Indicates Existence of Eight Conservative Social Psychologists," *Heterodox* (blog), January 7, 2016, https://heterodoxacademy .org/blog/new-study-indicates-existence-of-eight-conservative-social-psychol ogists/.

23 David Buss and William von Hippel, "Psychological Barriers to Evolutionary Psychology: Ideological Bias and Coalitional Adaptations," *Archives of Scientific Psychology* 6 (2018): 148–58, https://psycnet.apa.org/fulltext/2018-57934 -001.html.

24 Jay J. Van Bavel et al., "Breaking Groupthink: Why Scientific Identity and Norms Mitigate Ideological Epistemology," *Psychological Inquiry* 31, no. 1 (January 2, 2020): 66–72, https://doi.org/10.1080/1047840X.2020.1722599.

25 Diego Reinero et al., "Is the Political Slant of Psychology Research Related to Scientific Replicability?" (2019), https://doi.org/10.31234/osf.io/6k3j5.

26 Eitan, Orly, Domenico Viganola, Yoel Inbar, Anna Dreber, Magnus Johannes-son, Thomas Pfeiffer, Stefan Thau, and Eric Luis Uhlmann, "Is research in social psychology politically biased? Systematic empirical tests and a forecast-ing survey to address the controversy," *Journal of Experimental Social Psychology* 79 (2018): 188-99.

27 Niklas K. Steffens et al., "Our Followers Are Lions, Theirs Are Sheep: How Social Identity Shapes Theories about Followership and Social Influence," *Political Psychology* 39, no. 1 (2018): 23–42.

28 Packer, Ungson, and Marsh, "Conformity and Reactions to Deviance."

29 Gordon Pennycook et al., "Fighting COVID-19 Misinformation on Social Media: Experimental Evidence for a Scalable Accuracy-Nudge Interven-tion," *Psychological Science* 31, no. 7 (July 1, 2020): 770–80, https://doi.org /10.1177/0956797620939054.

CHAPTER 4: ESCAPING ECHO CHAMBERS

1 Dan M. Kahan et al., "Motivated Numeracy and Enlightened Self-Government," *Behavioural Public Policy* 1 (September 2013): 54–86, https://doi.org/10.2139 /ssrn.2319992.

2 Eli J. Finkel et al., "Political Sectarianism in America," *Science* 370, no. 6516 (October 30, 2020): 533–36, https://doi.org/10.1126/science.abe1715.

3 Elizabeth Ann Harris et al., "The Psychology and Neuroscience of Partisan-ship," PsyArXiv, October 13, 2020, https://doi.org/10.31234/osf.io /hdn2w.

4 Nick Rogers and Jason Jones, "Using Twitter Bios to Measure Changes in Social Identity: Are Americans Defining Themselves More Politically Over Time?" (August 2019), https://doi.org/10.13140/RG.2.2.32584.67849.

5 M. Keith Chen and Ryne Rohla, "The Effect of Partisanship and Political Ad-vertising on Close Family Ties," *Science* 360, no. 6392 (June 1, 2018): 1020–24, https://doi.org/10.1126/science.aaq1433.

6 Shanto Iyengar et al., "The Origins and Consequences of Affective Polariza-tion in the United States," *Annual Review of Political Science* 22, no. 1 (2019): 129–46, https://doi.org/10.1146/annurev-polisci-051117-073034.

7 Elaine Chen, "Group Think at the Inauguration?," *Only Human*, January 24,

2017, https://www.wnycstudios.org/podcasts/onlyhuman/articles/group-think -inauguration.

8 Finkel et al., "Political Sectarianism."

9 John R. Hibbing, Kevin B. Smith, and John R. Alford, *Predisposed: Liberals, Conservatives, and the Biology of Political Differences* (New York: Routledge, 2013).

10 Ryota Kanai et al., "Political Orientations Are Correlated with Brain Structure in Young Adults," *Current Biology* 21, no. 8 (April 26, 2011): 677–80, https://doi.org/10.1016/j.cub.2011.03.017.

11 H. Hannah Nam et al., "Amygdala Structure and the Tendency to Regard the Social System as Legitimate and Desirable," *Nature Human Behaviour* 2, no. 2 (February 2018): 133–38, https://doi.org/10.1038/s41562-017-0248-5.

12 H. Hannah Nam et al., "Toward a Neuropsychology of Political Orientation: Exploring Ideology in Patients with Frontal and Midbrain Lesions," *Philosophical Transactions of the Royal Society B: Biological Sciences* 376, no. 1822 (April 12, 2021): 20200137, https://doi.org/10.1098/rstb.2020.0137.

13 John T. Jost, Christopher M. Federico, and Jaime L. Napier, "Political Ideology: Its Structure, Functions, and Elective Affinities," *Annual Review of Psychology* 60, no. 1 (2009): 307–37, https://doi.org/10.1146/annurev.psych .60.110707.163600.

14 Dharshan Kumaran, Hans Ludwig Melo, and Emrah Duzel, "The Emergence and Representation of Knowledge About Social and Nonsocial Hierarchies," *Neuron* 76, no. 3 (November 8, 2012): 653–66, https://doi.org/10.1016 /j.neuron.2012.09.035.

15 Nam et al., "Amygdala Structure."

16 M. J. Crockett, "Moral Outrage in the Digital Age," *Nature Human Behaviour* 1, no. 11 (November 2017): 769–71, https://doi.org/10.1038/s41562-017 -0213-3.

17 Ibid.

18 "Average Person Scrolls 300 Feet of Social Media Content Daily," *NetNews-Ledger* (blog), January 1, 2018, http://www.netnewsledger.com/2018/01/01 /average-person-scrolls-300-feet-social-media-content-daily/.

19 William Brady, Ana Gantman, and Jay Van Bavel, "Attentional Capture Helps Explain Why Moral and Emotional Content Go Viral," *Journal of Experimental Psychology: General* 149 (September 5, 2019): 746–56, https://doi.org /10.1037/xge0000673.

20 Rich McCormick, "Donald Trump Says Facebook and Twitter 'Helped Him Win,'" *Verge*, November 13, 2016, https://www.theverge.com/2016/11/13 /13619148/trump-facebook-twitter-helped-win.

21 William J. Brady et al., "An Ideological Asymmetry in the Diffusion of Moralized Content Among Political Elites," PsyArXiv, September 28, 2018, https://doi.org/10.31234/osf.io/43n5e.

22 Marlon Mooijman et al., "Moralization in Social Networks and the Emergence of Violence During Protests," *Nature Human Behaviour* 2, no. 6 (2018): 389–96.

23 William J. Brady and Jay J. Van Bavel, "Social Identity Shapes Antecedents and Functional Outcomes of Moral Emotion Expression in Online Networks," OSF Preprints, April 2, 2021, https://doi:10.31219/osf.io/dgt6u.

24   Andrew M. Guess, Brendan Nyhan, and Jason Reifler, "Exposure to Untrust-
      worthy Websites in the 2016 US Election," *Nature Human Behaviour* 4, no. 5
      (May 2020): 472–80, https://doi.org/10.1038/s41562-020-0833-x.

25   Andrea Pereira, Jay J. Van Bavel, and Elizabeth Ann Harris, "Identity Con-
      cerns Drive Belief: The Impact of Partisan Identity on the Belief and
      Dissemination of True and False News," PsyArXiv, September 11, 2018,
      https://doi.org/10.31234/osf.io/7vc5d.

26   Mark Murray, "Sixty Percent Believe Worst Is Yet to Come for the U.S. in
      Coronavirus Pandemic," NBCNews.com, March 15, 2020, https://www
      .nbcnews.com/politics/meet-the-press/sixty-percent-believe-worst-yet-come
      -u-s-coronavirus-pandemic-n1159106.

27   Jay J. Van Bavel, "In a Pandemic, Political Polarization Could Kill People,"
      Washington Post, March 23, 2020, https://www.washingtonpost.com/outlook
      /2020/03/23/coronavirus-polarization-political-exaggeration/.

28   "Donald Trump, Charleston, South Carolina, Rally Transcript," *Rev* (blog),
      February 28, 2020, https://www.rev.com/blog/transcripts/donald-trump
      -charleston-south-carolina-rally-transcript-february-28-2020.

29   Anton Gollwitzer et al., "Partisan Differences in Physical Distancing Predict
      Infections and Mortality During the Coronavirus Pandemic," PsyArXiv, May
      24, 2020, https://doi.org/10.31234/osf.io/t3yxa.

30   Damien Cave, "Jacinda Ardern Sold a Drastic Lockdown with Straight Talk
      and Mom Jokes," *New York Times,* May 23, 2020, https://www.nytimes.com
      /2020/05/23/world/asia/jacinda-ardern-coronavirus-new-zealand.html.

31   David Levinsky, "Democrat Andy Kim Takes His Seat in Congress," *Burlington
      County Times,* January 3, 2019, https://www.burlingtoncountytimes.com
      /news/20190103/democrat-andy-kim-takes-his-seat-in-congress.

32   Bryce J. Dietrich, "Using Motion Detection to Measure Social Polarization in
      the U.S. House of Representatives," *Political Analysis* (November 2020): 1–10,
      https://doi.org/10.1017/pan.2020.25.

33   Christopher A. Bail et al., "Exposure to Opposing Views on Social Media Can
      Increase Political Polarization," *Proceedings of the National Academy of Sciences*
      115, no. 37 (September 11, 2018): 9216–21, https://doi.org/10.1073/pnas
      .1804840115.

34   Douglas Guilbeault, Joshua Becker, and Damon Centola, "Social Learning
      and Partisan Bias in the Interpretation of Climate Trends," *Proceedings of the
      National Academy of Sciences* 115, no. 39 (September 25, 2018): 9714–19,
      https://doi.org/10.1073/pnas.1722664115.

35   Erin Rossiter, "The Consequences of Interparty Conversation on Outparty
      Affect and Stereotypes," Washington University in St. Louis, September 4,
      2020, https://erossiter.com/files/conversations.pdf.

36   Hunt Allcott et al., "The Welfare Effects of Social Media," *American Economic
      Review* 119 (March 2020): 629–76, https://doi.org/10.1257/aer.20190658.

37   Abraham Rutchick, Joshua Smyth, and Sara Konrath, "Seeing Red (and
      Blue): Effects of Electoral College Depictions on Political Group Percep-
      tion," *Analyses of Social Issues and Public Policy* 9 (December 1, 2009): 269–82,
      https://doi.org/10.1111/j.1530-2415.2009.01183.x.

CHAPTER 5: THE VALUE OF IDENTITY

1   "What Is Truly Scandinavian?," Scandinavian Airlines, 2020, https://www
    .youtube.com/watch?v=ShfsBPrNcTI&ab_channel=SAS-ScandinavianAirlines.

2   "Nordic Airline SAS Criticised for Saying 'Absolutely Nothing' Is Truly Scan-
    dinavian," *Sky News,* February 14, 2020, https://news.sky.com/story/nordic
    -airline-sas-criticised-for-saying-absolutely-nothing-is-truly-scandinavian-11933
    757. Reaction to the ad was particularly negative among and may have been
    exacerbated by right-wing groups. The airline responded, "SAS is a
    Scandinavian airline that brings travelers to, from and within Scandinavia,
    and we stand behind the message in the film that travel enriches
    us...When we travel, we influence our surroundings and we are influenced
    by others."

3   "I Am Canadian—Best Commercial Ever!," CanadaWebDeveloper, April 2014,
    https://www.youtube.com/watch?v=pASE_TgeVg8&ab_channel=CanadaWeb
    Developer.

4   George A. Akerlof and Rachel E. Kranton, *Identity Economics: How Our Identi-
    ties Shape Our Work, Wages, and Well-Being* (Princeton, NJ: Princeton University
    Press, 2011).

5   "The Psychology of Stealing Office Supplies," BBC.com, May 24, 2018,
    https://www.bbc.com/worklife/article/20180524-the-psychology-of-stealing
    -office-supplies.

6   "Lukacs: Buckeyes Tradition 40 Years in the Making," ESPN.com, September
    12, 2008, https://www.espn.com/college-football/news/story?id=3583496.

7   "College Football's Winningest Teams over the Past 10 Years: Ranked!," *For the
    Win* (blog), August 19, 2015, https://ftw.usatoday.com/2015/08/best-college
    -football-teams-past-10-years-best-record-boise-state-ohio-state-most-wins.

8   Robert Cialdini et al., "Basking in Reflected Glory: Three (Football) Field Stud-
    ies," *Journal of Personality and Social Psychology* 34 (1976): 366–75,
    https://www.academia.edu/570635/Basking_in_reflected_glory_Three_foot
    ball_field_studies.

9   Leor M. Hackel, Jamil Zaki, and Jay J. Van Bavel, "Social Identity Shapes So-
    cial Valuation: Evidence from Prosocial Behavior and Vicarious Reward,"
    Social Cognitive and Affective Neuroscience 12, no. 8 (August 1, 2017): 1219–28,
    https://doi.org/10.1093/scan/nsx045.

10 Robert D. Putnam, *Bowling Alone: The Collapse and Revival of American Commu-
    nity* (New York: Simon and Schuster, 2000).

11 Kurt Hugenberg et al., "The Categorization-Individuation Model: An Inte-
    grative Account of the Other-Race Recognition Deficit," *Psychological Review*
    117, no. 4 (2010): 1168.

12 Jay J. Van Bavel et al., "Motivated Social Memory: Belonging Needs Moderate
    the Own-Group Bias in Face Recognition," *Journal of Experimental Social Psy-
    chology* 48, no. 3 (2012): 707–13.

13 Katherine E. Loveland, Dirk Smeesters, and Naomi Mandel, "Still Preoccu-
    pied with 1995: The Need to Belong and Preference for Nostalgic Products,"
    Journal of Consumer Research 37, no. 3 (2010): 393–408.

14 Maya D. Guendelman, Sapna Cheryan, and Benoît Monin, "Fitting In but
    Getting Fat: Identity Threat and Dietary Choices Among U.S. Immigrant

Groups," *Psychological Science* 22, no. 7 (July 1, 2011): 959–67, https://doi.org/10.1177/0956797611411585.

15 Marilynn B. Brewer, "The Social Self: On Being the Same and Different at the Same Time," *Personality and Social Psychology Bulletin* 17, no. 5 (October 1, 1991): 475–82, https://doi.org/10.1177/0146167291175001.

16 Karl Taeuscher, Ricarda B. Bouncken, and Robin Pesch, "Gaining Legitimacy by Being Different: Optimal Distinctiveness in Crowdfunding Platforms," *Academy of Management Journal* 64, no. 1 (2020): 149–79.

17 Steven E. Sexton and Alison L. Sexton, "Conspicuous Conservation: The Prius Halo and Willingness to Pay for Environmental Bona Fides," *Journal of Environmental Economics and Management* 67, no. 3 (2014): 303–17.

18 Rachel Greenspan, "Lori Loughlin and Felicity Huffman's College Admissions Scandal Remains Ongoing," *Time*, March 3, 2019, https://time.com/5549921/college-admissions-bribery-scandal/.

19 Paul Rozin et al., "Asymmetrical Social Mach Bands: Exaggeration of Social Identities on the More Esteemed Side of Group Borders," *Psychological Science* 25, no. 10 (2014): 1955–59.

20 Cindy Harmon-Jones, Brandon J. Schmeichel, and Eddie Harmon-Jones, "Symbolic Self-Completion in Academia: Evidence from Department Web Pages and Email Signature Files," *European Journal of Social Psychology* 39 (2009): 311–16.

21 Robert A. Wicklund and Peter M. Gollwitzer, "Symbolic Self-Completion, Attempted Influence, and Self-Deprecation," *Basic and Applied Social Psychology* 2, no. 2 (June 1981): 89–114, https://doi.org/10.1207/s15324834basp0202_2.

22 Margaret Foddy, Michael J. Platow, and Toshio Yamagishi, "Group-Based Trust in Strangers: The Role of Stereotypes and Expectations," *Psychological Science* 20, no. 4 (April 1, 2009): 419–22, https://doi.org/10.1111/j.1467-9280.2009.02312.x.

23 Toshio Yamagishi and Toko Kiyonari, "The Group as the Container of Generalized Reciprocity," *Social Psychology Quarterly* 63, no. 2 (2000): 116–32, https://doi.org/10.2307/2695887.

CHAPTER 6: OVERCOMING BIAS

1 Chris Palmer and Stephanie Farr, "Philly Police Dispatcher After 911 Call: 'Group of Males' Was 'Causing a Disturbance' at Starbucks," *Philadelphia Inquirer*, April 17, 2018, https://www.inquirer.com/philly/news/crime/philly-police-release-audio-of-911-call-from-philadelphia-starbucks-20180417.html; "Starbucks to Close All U.S. Stores for Racial-Bias Education," Starbucks.com, April 17, 2018, https://stories.starbucks.com/press/2018/starbucks-to-close-stores-nationwide-for-racial-bias-education-may-29/; Samantha Melamed, "Starbucks Arrests in Philadelphia: CEO Kevin Johnson Promises Unconscious-Bias Training for Managers," *Philadelphia Inquirer*, April 16, 2018, https://www.inquirer.com/philly/news/pennsylvania/philadelphia/starbucks-ceo-kevin-johnson-philadelphia-arrests-black-men-20180416.html.

2 "Subverting Starbucks," *Newsweek*, October 27, 2002, https://www.newsweek.com/subverting-starbucks-146749.

Notes

Notes

Notes

3 Rob Tornoe, "What Happened at Starbucks in Philadelphia?," *Philadelphia Inquirer*, April 16, 2018, https://www.inquirer.com/philly/news/starbucks philadelphia-arrests-black-men-video-viral-protests-background-20180416.html.
4 "Starbucks to Close All U.S. Stores." https://stories.starbucks.com/press /2018/starbucks-to-close-stores-nationwide-for-racial-bias-education-may-29.
5 Mahzarin R. Banaji and Anthony G. Greenwald, *Blindspot: Hidden Biases of Good People* (New York: Bantam, 2016); Bertram Gawronski and Jan De Houwer, "Implicit Measures in Social and Personality Psychology," in *Handbook of Research Methods in Social and Personality Psychology*, ed. Harry Reis and Charles Judd (New York: Cambridge University Press, 2014).
6 Po Bronson, "Is Your Baby Racist?," *Newsweek*, September 6, 2009, https://www .newsweek.com/nurtureshock-cover-story-newsweek-your-baby-racist-223434.
7 Leda Cosmides, John Tooby, and Robert Kurzban, "Perceptions of Race," *Trends in Cognitive Sciences* 7, no. 4 (2003): 173–79.
8 Donald E. Brown, "Human Universals, Human Nature and Human Culture," *Daedalus* 133, no. 4 (2004): 47–54.
9 Jim Sidanius and Felicia Pratto, *Social Dominance: An Intergroup Theory of Social Hierarchy and Oppression* (New York: Cambridge University Press, 2001).
10 Gunnar Myrdal, *An American Dilemma*, vol. 2 (Rutgers, NJ: Transaction Publishers, 1996).
11 Nathan Nunn, "Slavery, Inequality, and Economic Development in the Americas," *Institutions and Economic Performance* 15 (2008): 148–80; Nathan Nunn, "The Historical Roots of Economic Development," *Science* 367, no. 6485 (2020).
12 Avidit Acharya, Matthew Blackwell, and Maya Sen, "The Political Legacy of American Slavery," *Journal of Politics* 78, no. 3 (2016): 621–41.
13 B. Keith Payne, Heidi A. Vuletich, and Kristjen B. Lundberg, "The Bias of Crowds: How Implicit Bias Bridges Personal and Systemic Prejudice," *Psychological Inquiry* 28, no. 4 (2017): 233–48.
14 Rachel Treisman, "Nearly 100 Confederate Monuments Removed in 2020, Report Says; More than 700 Remain," National Public Radio, February 23, 2021, https://www.npr.org/2021/02/23/970610428/nearly-100-confederate -monuments-removed-in-2020-report-says-more-than-700-remai.
15 Elizabeth A. Phelps et al., "Performance on Indirect Measures of Race Evaluation Predicts Amygdala Activation," *Journal of Cognitive Neuroscience* 12, no. 5 (2000): 729–38.
16 William A. Cunningham et al., "Separable Neural Components in the Processing of Black and White Faces," *Psychological Science* 15, no. 12 (2004): 806–13.
17 Jay J. Van Bavel, Dominic J. Packer, and William A. Cunningham, "The Neural Substrates of In-Group Bias: A Functional Magnetic Resonance Imaging Investigation," *Psychological Science* 19, no. 11 (2008): 1131–39.
18 Ibid.; Jay J. Van Bavel and William A. Cunningham, "Self-Categorization with a Novel Mixed-Race Group Moderates Automatic Social and Racial Biases," *Personality and Social Psychology Bulletin* 35, no. 3 (2009): 321–35; Jay J. Van Bavel and William A. Cunningham, "A Social Identity Approach to Person Memory: Group Membership, Collective Identification, and Social Role Shape Attention and Memory," *Personality and Social Psychology Bulletin* 38, no. 12 (2012): 1566–78.
19 João F. Guassi Moreira, Jay J. Van Bavel, and Eva H. Telzer, "The Neural De-

288

velopment of 'Us and Them,'" *Social Cognitive and Affective Neuroscience* 12, no. 2 (2017): 184–96.

20 Anthony W. Scroggins et al., "Reducing Prejudice with Labels: Shared Group Memberships Attenuate Implicit Bias and Expand Implicit Group Boundaries," *Personality and Social Psychology Bulletin* 42, no. 2 (2016): 219–29.

21 Calvin K. Lai et al., "Reducing Implicit Racial Preferences: I. A Comparative Investigation of 17 Interventions," *Journal of Experimental Psychology: General* 143, no. 4 (2014): 1765.

22 Salma Mousa, "Building Social Cohesion Between Christians and Muslims Through Soccer in Post-ISIS Iraq," *Science* 369, no. 6505 (2020): 866–70.

23 Ala' Alrababa'h et al., "Can Exposure to Celebrities Reduce Prejudice? The Effect of Mohamed Salah on Islamophobic Behaviors and Attitudes," *American Political Science Review* (2021): 1–18.

24 Emma Pierson et al., "A Large-Scale Analysis of Racial Disparities in Police Stops Across the United States," *Nature Human Behaviour* 4, no. 7 (July 2020): 736–45, https://doi.org/10.1038/s41562-020-0858-1.

25 Keith Barry and Andy Bergmann, "The Crash Test Bias: How Male-Focused Testing Puts Female Drivers at Risk," *Consumer Reports*, October 23, 2019, https://www.consumerreports.org/car-safety/crash-test-bias-how-male-focused-testing-puts-female-drivers-at-risk/.

26 Deborah Vagins and Jesselyn McCurdy, "Cracks in the System: 20 Years of the Unjust Federal Crack Cocaine Law," American Civil Liberties Union, October 2006, https://www.aclu.org/other/cracks-system-20-years-unjust-federal-crack-cocaine-law.

27 Julia Stoyanovich, Jay J. Van Bavel, and Tessa V. West, "The Imperative of Interpretable Machines," *Nature Machine Intelligence* 2, no. 4 (2020): 197–99.

28 Katrine Berg Nødtvedt et al., "Racial Bias in the Sharing Economy and the Role of Trust and Self-Congruence," *Journal of Experimental Psychology: General* (February 2021).

29 Lynne G. Zucker, "Production of Trust: Institutional Sources of Economic Structure, 1840–1920," *Research in Organizational Behavior* (1986): 53–111; Delia Baldassarri and Maria Abascal, "Diversity and Prosocial Behavior," *Science* 369, no. 6508 (2020): 1183–87.

30 Shiang-Yi Lin and Dominic J. Packer, "Dynamic Tuning of Evaluations: Implicit Racial Attitudes Are Sensitive to Incentives for Intergroup Cooperation," *Social Cognition* 35, no. 3 (2017): 245–72.

CHAPTER 7: FINDING SOLIDARITY

1 Sylvia R. Jacobson, "Individual and Group Responses to Confinement in a Skyjacked Plane," *American Journal of Orthopsychiatry* 43, no. 3 (1973): 459.

2 Ibid.

3 Martin Gansberg, "37 Who Saw Murder Didn't Call the Police," *New York Times*, March 27, 1964, https://www.nytimes.com/1964/03/27/archives/37-who-saw-murder-didnt-call-the-police-apathy-at-stabbing-of.html.

4 Mark Levine, "Helping in Emergencies: Revisiting Latané and Darley's Bystander Studies," in *Social Psychology: Revisiting the Classic Studies*, ed. J. R.

Smith and S. A. Haslam (Thousand Oaks, CA: Sage Publications, 2012), 192–208.

5   Bibb Latané and John M. Darley, "Group Inhibition of Bystander Intervention in Emergencies," *Journal of Personality and Social Psychology* 10, no. 3 (1968): 215.

6   Levine, "Helping in Emergencies."

7   Richard Philpot et al., "Would I Be Helped? Cross-National CCTV Footage Shows That Intervention Is the Norm in Public Conflicts," *American Psychologist* 75, no. 1 (2020): 66.

8   Peter Fischer et al., "The Bystander-Effect: A Meta-Analytic Review on Bystander Intervention in Dangerous and Non-Dangerous Emergencies," *Psychological Bulletin* 137, no. 4 (2011): 517.

9   Peter Singer, *The Expanding Circle: Ethics, Evolution, and Moral Progress* (Princeton, NJ: Princeton University Press, 2011).

10 Mark Levine et al., "Identity and Emergency Intervention: How Social Group Membership and Inclusiveness of Group Boundaries Shape Helping Behavior," *Personality and Social Psychology Bulletin* 31, no. 4 (2005): 443–53.

11 John Drury et al., "Facilitating Collective Psychosocial Resilience in the Public in Emergencies: Twelve Recommendations Based on the Social Identity Approach," *Frontiers in Public Health* 7 (2019): 141; John Drury, "The Role of Social Identity Processes in Mass Emergency Behaviour: An Integrative Review," *European Review of Social Psychology* 29, no. 1 (2018): 38–81; John Drury, Chris Cocking, and Steve Reicher, "The Nature of Collective Resilience: Survivor Reactions to the 2005 London Bombings," *International Journal of Mass Emergencies and Disasters* 27, no. 1 (2009): 66–95.

12 Drury, Cocking, and Reicher, "The Nature of Collective Resilience."

13 Diego A. Reinero, Suzanne Dikker, and Jay J. Van Bavel, "Inter-Brain Synchrony in Teams Predicts Collective Performance," *Social Cognitive and Affective Neuroscience* 16, nos. 1–2 (2021): 43–57.

14 Suzanne Dikker et al., "Brain-to-Brain Synchrony Tracks Real-World Dynamic Group Interactions in the Classroom," *Current Biology* 27, no. 9 (2017): 1375–80.

15 Jackson Katz, *Macho Paradox: Why Some Men Hurt Women and How All Men Can Help* (Napierville, IL: Sourcebooks, 2006).

16 Henri Tajfel and John Turner, "An Integrative Theory of Intergroup Conflict," *Social Psychology of Intergroup Relations* 33 (1979); B. Bettencourt et al., "Status Differences and In-Group Bias: A Meta-Analytic Examination of the Effects of Status Stability, Status Legitimacy, and Group Permeability," *Psychological Bulletin* 127, no. 4 (2001): 520.

17 John T. Jost and Mahzarin R. Banaji, "The Role of Stereotyping in System-Justification and the Production of False Consciousness," *British Journal of Social Psychology* 33, no. 1 (1994): 1–27; Aaron C. Kay and Justin Friesen, "On Social Stability and Social Change: Understanding When System Justification Does and Does Not Occur," *Current Directions in Psychological Science* 20, no. 6 (2011): 360–64.

18 Kees Van den Bos and Marjolein Maas, "On the Psychology of the Belief in a Just World: Exploring Experiential and Rationalistic Paths to Victim Blaming," *Personality and Social Psychology Bulletin* 35, no. 12 (2009): 1567–78; Bernard Weiner, Danny Osborne, and Udo Rudolph, "An Attributional Ana-

lysis of Reactions to Poverty: The Political Ideology of the Giver and the Perceived Morality of the Receiver," *Personality and Social Psychology Review* 15, no. 2 (2011): 199–213.

19   Kelly Danaher and Nyla R. Branscombe, "Maintaining the System with Tokenism: Bolstering Individual Mobility Beliefs and Identification with a Discriminatory Organization," *British Journal of Social Psychology* 49, no. 2 (2010): 343–62.

20   Cheryl R. Kaiser et al., "The Ironic Consequences of Obama's Election: Decreased Support for Social Justice," *Journal of Experimental Social Psychology* 45, no. 3 (2009): 556–59.

21   Amy R. Krosch et al., "On the Ideology of Hypodescent: Political Conservatism Predicts Categorization of Racially Ambiguous Faces as Black," *Journal of Experimental Social Psychology* 49, no. 6 (2013): 1196–1203; Jojanneke Van der Toorn et al., "In Defense of Tradition: Religiosity, Conservatism, and Opposition to Same-Sex Marriage in North America," *Personality and Social Psychology Bulletin* 43, no. 10 (2017): 1455–68.

22   "Protesters' Anger Justified Even if Actions May Not Be," Monmouth University Polling Institute, June 2, 2020, https://www.monmouth.edu/polling -institute/reports/monmouthpoll_us_060220/.

23   Emina Subašić et al., " 'We for She': Mobilising Men and Women to Act in Solidarity for Gender Equality," *Group Processes and Intergroup Relations* 21, no. 5 (2018): 707–24; Emina Subašić, Katherine J. Reynolds, and John C. Turner, "The Political Solidarity Model of Social Change: Dynamics of Self-Categorization in Intergroup Power Relations," *Personality and Social Psychology Review* 12, no. 4 (2008): 330–52.

24   John Drury et al., "A Social Identity Model of Riot Diffusion: From Injustice to Empowerment in the 2011 London Riots," *European Journal of Social Psychology* 50, no. 3 (2020): 646–61; Cliff Stott and Steve Reicher, *Mad Mobs and Englishmen? Myths and Realities of the 2011 Riots* (London: Constable and Robinson, 2011).

25   John Drury et al., "Re-Reading the 2011 English Riots—ESRC 'Beyond Contagion' Interim Report," January 2019, https://sro.sussex.ac.uk/id/eprint/82292 /1/Re-reading%20the%202011%20riots%20ESRC%20Beyond%20Contagion %20interim%20report.pdf.

26   Stephen Reicher et al., "An Integrated Approach to Crowd Psychology and Public Order Policing," *Policing* 27 (December 2004): 558–72; Clifford Stott and Matthew Radburn, "Understanding Crowd Conflict: Social Context, Psychology and Policing," *Current Opinion in Psychology* 35 (March 2020): 76–80.

27   Maria J. Stephan and Erica Chenoweth, "Why Civil Resistance Works: The Strategic Logic of Nonviolent Conflict," *International Security* 33, no. 1 (2008): 7–44; Erica Chenoweth and Maria J. Stephan, *Why Civil Resistance Works: The Strategic Logic of Nonviolent Conflict* (New York: Columbia University Press, 2011).

28   Matthew Feinberg, Robb Willer, and Chloe Kovacheff, "The Activist's Dilemma: Extreme Protest Actions Reduce Popular Support for Social Movements," *Journal of Personality and Social Psychology* 119 (2020): 1086–111.

29   Omar Wasow, "Agenda Seeding: How 1960s Black Protests Moved Elites, Public Opinion and Voting," *American Political Science Review* 114, no. 3 (2020): 638–59.

CHAPTER 8: FOSTERING DISSENT

1   Lily Rothman, "Read the Letter That Changed the Way Americans Saw the Vietnam War," *Time*, March 16, 2015, https://time.com/3732062/ronald-ridenhour-vietnam-my-lai/; John H. Cushman Jr, "Ronald Ridenhour, 52, Veteran Who Reported My Lai Massacre," *New York Times*, May 11, 1998, https://www.nytimes.com/1998/05/11/us/ronald-ridenhour-52-veteran-who-reported-my-lai-massacre.html.

2   Ron Ridenhour, "Ridenhour Letter," http://www.digitalhistory.uh.edu/active_learning/explorations/vietnam/ridenhour_letter.cfm.

3   Ronald L. Ridenhour, "One Man's Bitter Porridge," *New York Times*, November 10, 1973, https://www.nytimes.com/1973/11/10/archives/one-mans-bitter-porridge.html.

4   Jeffrey Jones, "Americans Divided on Whether King's Dream Has Been Realized," Gallup.com, August 26, 2011, https://news.gallup.com/poll/149201/Americans-Divided-Whether-King-Dream-Realized.aspx.

5   Benoît Monin, Pamela J. Sawyer, and Matthew J. Marquez, "The Rejection of Moral Rebels: Resenting Those Who Do the Right Thing," *Journal of Personality and Social Psychology* 95, no. 1 (2008): 76; Kieran O'Connor and Benoît Monin, "When Principled Deviance Becomes Moral Threat: Testing Alternative Mechanisms for the Rejection of Moral Rebels," *Group Processes and Intergroup Relations* 19, no. 5 (2016): 676–93.

6   Craig D. Parks and Asako B. Stone, "The Desire to Expel Unselfish Members from the Group," *Journal of Personality and Social Psychology* 99, no. 2 (2010): 303.

7   Jasmine Tata et al., "Proportionate Group Size and Rejection of the Deviate: A Meta-Analytic Integration," *Journal of Social Behavior and Personality* 11, no. 4 (1996): 739.

8   José Marques, Dominic Abrams, and Rui G. Serôdio, "Being Better by Being Right: Subjective Group Dynamics and Derogation of In-Group Deviants When Generic Norms Are Undermined," *Journal of Personality and Social Psychology* 81, no. 3 (2001): 436; Arie W. Kruglanski and Donna M. Webster, "Group Members' Reactions to Opinion Deviates and Conformists at Varying Degrees of Proximity to Decision Deadline and of Environmental Noise," *Journal of Personality and Social Psychology* 61, no. 2 (1991): 212; Matthew J. Hornsey, "Dissent and Deviance in Intergroup Contexts," *Current Opinion in Psychology* 11 (2016): 1–5.

9   Charlan J. Nemeth and Jack A. Goncalo, "Rogues and Heroes: Finding Value in Dissent," in *Rebels in Groups: Dissent, Deviance, Difference, and Defiance*, ed. Jolanda Jetten and Matthew Hornsey (Chichester, UK: Wiley-Blackwell, 2011), 17–35; Charlan Jeanne Nemeth and Joel Wachtler, "Creative Problem Solving as a Result of Majority vs. Minority Influence," *European Journal of Social Psychology* 13, no. 1 (1983): 45–55.

10 Linn Van Dyne and Richard Saavedra, "A Naturalistic Minority Influence Experiment: Effects on Divergent Thinking, Conflict and Originality in Work-Groups," *British Journal of Social Psychology* 35, no. 1 (1996): 151–67.

11 Randall S. Peterson et al., "Group Dynamics in Top Management Teams: Groupthink, Vigilance, and Alternative Models of Organizational Failure and

Success," *Organizational Behavior and Human Decision Processes* 73, nos. 2–3 (1998): 272–305.

12   Codou Samba, Daan Van Knippenberg, and C. Chet Miller, "The Impact of Strategic Dissent on Organizational Outcomes: A Meta-Analytic Integration," *Strategic Management Journal* 39, no. 2 (2018): 379–402.

13   Ibid.

14   Solomon E. Asch, "Opinions and Social Pressure," *Scientific American* 193, no. 5 (1955): 31–35; Solomon E. Asch, "Studies of Independence and Conformity: I. A Minority of One Against a Unanimous Majority," *Psychological Monographs: General and Applied* 70, no. 9 (1956): 1–70.

15   Stanley Milgram, "Behavioral Study of Obedience," *Journal of Abnormal and Social Psychology* 67, no. 4 (1963): 371; Stanley Milgram, *Obedience to Authority* (New York: Harper and Row, 1974).

16   Dominic J. Packer, "Identifying Systematic Disobedience in Milgram's Obedience Experiments: A Meta-Analytic Review," *Perspectives on Psychological Science* 3, no. 4 (2008): 301–4; Jerry M. Burger, "Replicating Milgram: Would People Still Obey Today?," *American Psychologist* 64, no. 1 (2009): 1.

17   Stephen D. Reicher, S. Alexander Haslam, and Joanne R. Smith, "Working Toward the Experimenter: Reconceptualizing Obedience Within the Milgram Paradigm as Identification-Based Followership," *Perspectives on Psychological Science* 7, no. 4 (2012): 315–24.

18   Bert H. Hodges et al., "Speaking from Ignorance: Not Agreeing with Others We Believe Are Correct," *Journal of Personality and Social Psychology* 106, no. 2 (2014): 218; Bert H. Hodges and Anne L. Geyer, "A Nonconformist Account of the Asch Experiments: Values, Pragmatics, and Moral Dilemmas," *Personality and Social Psychology Review* 10, no. 1 (2006): 2–19.

19   Dominic J. Packer, "On Being Both with Us and Against Us: A Normative Conflict Model of Dissent in Social Groups," *Personality and Social Psychology Review* 12, no. 1 (2008): 50–72; Dominic J. Packer and Christopher T. H. Miners, "Tough Love: The Normative Conflict Model and a Goal System Approach to Dissent Decisions," *Social and Personality Psychology Compass* 8, no. 7 (2014): 354–73.

20   Dominic J. Packer, Kentaro Fujita, and Alison L. Chasteen, "The Motivational Dynamics of Dissent Decisions: A Goal-Conflict Approach," *Social Psychological and Personality Science* 5, no. 1 (2014): 27–34.

21   Ibid.

22   Darcy R. Dupuis et al., "To Dissent and Protect: Stronger Collective Identification Increases Willingness to Dissent When Group Norms Evoke Collective Angst," *Group Processes and Intergroup Relations* 19, no. 5 (2016): 694–710.

23   Dominic J. Packer, "The Interactive Influence of Conscientiousness and Openness to Experience on Dissent," *Social Influence* 5, no. 3 (2010): 202–19.

24   Amy C. Edmondson, "Speaking Up in the Operating Room: How Team Leaders Promote Learning in Interdisciplinary Action Teams," *Journal of Management Studies* 40, no. 6 (2003): 1419–52.

25   Amy C. Edmondson and Zhike Lei, "Psychological Safety: The History, Renaissance, and Future of an Interpersonal Construct," *Annual Review of Organizational Psychology and Organizational Behavior* 1, no. 1 (2014): 23–43.

26   Charles Duhigg, "What Google Learned from Its Quest to Build the Perfect

Team," *Sunday New York Times Magazine*, February 25, 2016, https://www
.nytimes.com/2016/02/28/magazine/what-google-learned-from-its-quest
-to-build-the-perfect-team.html.

27 American Foreign Service Association, "Constructive Dissent Awards," 2019,
https://www.afsa.org/constructive-dissent-awards.

28 Monin, Sawyer, and Marquez, "The Rejection of Moral Rebels"; Alexander
H. Jordan and Benoît Monin, "From Sucker to Saint: Moralization in Response to Self-Threat," *Psychological Science* 19, no. 8 (2008): 809–15.

CHAPTER 9: LEADING EFFECTIVELY

1 Sinéad Baker, "'We're Just Having a Bit of an Earthquake Here': New Zealand's Jacinda Ardern Was Unfazed When an Earthquake Hit during a Live
Interview," *Business Insider*, May 25, 2020, https://www.businessinsider
.com.au/earthquake-interrupts-jacinda-ardern-in-live-interview-new-zealand
-2020-5.

2 Michelle Mark, "Iconic Photo of Boy Feeling Obama's Hair Was Taken 10
Years Ago," *Insider*, May 9, 2019, https://www.insider.com/photo-of-boy
-feeling-obamas-hair-taken-10-years-ago-2019-5.

3 Howard E. Gardner, *Leading Minds: An Anatomy of Leadership* (New York: Basic
Books, 1995).

4 Taylor Branch, *Parting the Waters: America in the King Years 1954–63* (New York:
Simon and Schuster, 2007).

5 Henry Mintzberg, *Mintzberg on Management: Inside Our Strange World of Organizations* (New York: Simon and Schuster, 1989).

6, "Truman Quotes," *Truman Library Institute* (blog), 2021, https://www
.trumanlibraryinstitute.org/truman/truman-quotes/.

7 Julian Barling, *The Science of Leadership: Lessons from Research for Organizational
Leaders* (New York: Oxford University Press, 2014).

8 Xiao-Hua Frank Wang and Jane M. Howell, "Exploring the Dual-Level Effects
of Transformational Leadership on Followers," *Journal of Applied Psychology* 95,
no. 6 (2010): 1134; Xiao-Hua Frank Wang and Jane M. Howell, "A Multilevel
Study of Transformational Leadership, Identification, and Follower Outcomes," *Leadership Quarterly* 23, no. 5 (2012): 775–90.

9 Niall O'Dowd, "Mary Robinson, the Woman Who Changed Ireland," *Irish Central*, March 8, 2021, https://www.irishcentral.com/opinion/nialloddowd/mary
-robinson-woman-changed-ireland.

10 "Address by the President, Mary Robinson, on the Occasion of Her Inauguration as President of Ireland," Office of the President of Ireland, December 3,
1990, https://president.ie/index.php/en/media-library/speeches/address
-by-the-president-mary-robinson-on-the-occasion-of-her-inauguration.

11 Viviane Seyranian and Michelle C. Bligh, "Presidential Charismatic Leadership: Exploring the Rhetoric of Social Change," *Leadership Quarterly* 19, no. 1
(2008): 54–76.

12 Niklas K. Steffens and S. Alexander Haslam, "Power Through 'Us': Leaders'
Use of We-Referencing Language Predicts Election Victory," *PLOS ONE* 8, no.
10 (2013): e77952; Martin P. Fladerer et al., "The Value of Speaking for 'Us':

The Relationship Between CEOs' Use of I- and We-Referencing Language and Subsequent Organizational Performance," *Journal of Business and Psychology* 36, no. 2 (April 2021): 299–313, https://doi.org/10.1007/s10869-019 -09677-0.

13   Leon Festinger, Henry Riecken, and Stanley Schachter, *When Prophecy Fails* (New York: Harper and Row, 1964).

14   Roderick M. Kramer, "Responsive Leaders: Cognitive and Behavioral Reactions to Identity Threats," in *Social Psychology and Organizations,* ed. David De Cremer, Rolf van Dick, and J. Keith Murnighan (New York: Routledge, 2011).

15   Kimberly D. Elsbach and Roderick M. Kramer, "Members' Responses to Organizational Identity Threats: Encountering and Countering the *Business Week* Rankings," *Administrative Science Quarterly* 41 (1996): 442–76.

16   Ibid.

17   David De Cremer and Tom R. Tyler, "On Being the Leader and Acting Fairly: A Contingency Approach," in *Social Psychology and Organizations,* ed. David De Cremer, Rolf van Dick, and J. Keith Murnighan (New York: Routledge, 2011).

18   Kurt T. Dirks, "Trust in Leadership and Team Performance: Evidence from NCAA Basketball," *Journal of Applied Psychology* 85, no. 6 (2000): 1004.

19   Ibid.

20   S. Alexander Haslam, Stephen D. Reicher, and Michael J. Platow, *The New Psychology of Leadership: Identity, Influence and Power* (New York: Routledge, 2020); Michael A. Hogg, "A Social Identity Theory of Leadership," *Personality and Social Psychology Review* 5, no. 3 (2001): 184–200.

21   Ashleigh Shelby Rosette, Geoffrey J. Leonardelli, and Katherine W. Phillips, "The White Standard: Racial Bias in Leader Categorization," *Journal of Applied Psychology* 93, no. 4 (2008): 758.

22   David E. Rast III, "Leadership in Times of Uncertainty: Recent Findings, Debates, and Potential Future Research Directions," *Social and Personality Psychology Compass* 9, no. 3 (2015): 133–45.

23   Michelle K. Ryan and S. Alexander Haslam, "The Glass Cliff: Evidence That Women Are Over-Represented in Precarious Leadership Positions," *British Journal of Management* 16, no. 2 (2005): 81–90; Michelle K. Ryan et al., "Getting on Top of the Glass Cliff: Reviewing a Decade of Evidence, Explanations, and Impact," *Leadership Quarterly* 27, no. 3 (2016): 446–55; Alison Cook and Christy Glass, "Above the Glass Ceiling: When Are Women and Racial/Ethnic Minorities Promoted to CEO?," *Strategic Management Journal* 35, no. 7 (2014): 1080–89.

24   Tom R. Tyler and E. Allan Lind, "A Relational Model of Authority in Groups," *Advances in Experimental Social Psychology* 25 (1992): 115–91.

25   Daan Van Knippenberg, "Leadership and Identity," in *The Nature of Leadership,* 2nd ed., ed. David Day and John Antonakis (London: Sage, 2012).

26   Robert A. Burgelman and Andrew S. Grove, "Strategic Dissonance," *California Management Review* 38, no. 2 (1996): 8–28.

27   Martin Gilbert, "I Shall Be the One to Save London," *Churchill Project* (blog), April 14, 2017, https://winstonchurchill.hillsdale.edu/shall-one-save-london/.

28   Andrew Roberts, *Churchill: Walking with Destiny* (New York: Penguin, 2018); Erik Larson, *The Splendid and the Vile: A Saga of Churchill, Family, and Defiance During the Blitz* (New York: Crown, 2020).

29 Roderick M. Kramer, "The Imperatives of Identity: The Role of Identity in Leader Judgment and Decision Making," in *Leadership and Power: Identity Processes in Groups and Organizations*, ed. Daan Van Knippenberg and Michael A. Hogg (London: Sage, 2003), 184.

30 Blake Ashforth, "Petty Tyranny in Organizations," *Human Relations* 47, no. 7 (1994): 755–78.

31 Birgit Schyns and Jan Schilling, "How Bad Are the Effects of Bad Leaders? A Meta-Analysis of Destructive Leadership and Its Outcomes," *Leadership Quarterly* 24, no. 1 (2013): 138–58.

32 Craig Haney, W. Curtis Banks, and Philip G. Zimbardo, "A Study of Prisoners and Guards in a Simulated Prison," *Naval Research Reviews* 9, nos. 1–17 (1973); "The Mind Is a Formidable Jailer," *New York Times,* April 8, 1973, https://www.nytimes.com/1973/04/08/archives/a-pirandellian-prison-the-mind-is-a-formidable-jailer.html; "Stanford Prison Experiment," https://www.prisonexp.org.

33 Philip G. Zimbardo, *The Lucifer Effect: Understanding How Good People Turn Evil* (New York: Random House, 2007).

34 S. Alexander Haslam and Stephen D. Reicher, "When Prisoners Take over the Prison: A Social Psychology of Resistance," *Personality and Social Psychology Review* 16, no. 2 (2012): 154–79; Stephen Reicher and S. Alexander Haslam, "Rethinking the Psychology of Tyranny: The BBC Prison Study," *British Journal of Social Psychology* 45, no. 1 (2006): 1–40; S. Alexander Haslam, Stephen D. Reicher, and Jay J. Van Bavel, "Rethinking the Nature of Cruelty: The Role of Identity Leadership in the Stanford Prison Experiment," *American Psychologist* 74, no. 7 (2019): 809.

35 Haslam, Reicher, and Van Bavel, "Rethinking the Nature of Cruelty." Stanford University Libraries (2018). Interviews from the Stanford Prison Experiment (audio recording; Source ID: SC0750_s5_b2_21). http://purl.stanford.edu/wn708sq0050.

36 Stephen Reicher, S. Alexander Haslam, and Rakshi Rath, "Making a Virtue of Evil: A Five-Step Social Identity Model of the Development of Collective Hate," *Social and Personality Psychology Compass* 2, no. 3 (2008): 1313–44.

37 Robert O. Paxton, *The Anatomy of Fascism* (New York: Vintage, 2007).

CHAPTER 10: THE FUTURE OF IDENTITY

1 William Ewald, ed., *Environment and Change: The Next Fifty Years* (Bloomington: Indiana University Press, 1968).

2 Herman Kahn and Anthony Wiener, "Faustian Powers and Human Choices: Some Twenty-First Century Technological and Economic Issues," in ibid.

3 *World Social Report 2020: Inequality in a Rapidly Changing World* (United Nations, February 2020), https://doi.org/10.18356/7f5d0efc-en.

4 Keith Payne, *The Broken Ladder: How Inequality Affects the Way We Think, Live, and Die* (New York: Penguin, 2017); Richard Wilkinson and Kate Pickett, *The Spirit Level: Why Greater Equality Makes Societies Stronger* (New York: Bloomsbury, 2011).

5 Niklas K. Steffens et al., "Identity Economics Meets Identity Leadership: Ex-

ploring the Consequences of Elevated CEO Pay," *Leadership Quarterly* 30 (June 2020).

6   Mark Rubin and Rebecca Stuart, "Kill or Cure? Different Types of Social Class Identification Amplify and Buffer the Relation Between Social Class and Mental Health," *Journal of Social Psychology* 158, no. 2 (2018): 236–51.

7   Frank Mols and Jolanda Jetten, *The Wealth Paradox: Economic Prosperity and the Hardening of Attitudes* (New York: Cambridge University Press, 2017); Frank Mols and Jolanda Jetten, "Explaining the Appeal of Populist Right-Wing Parties in Times of Economic Prosperity," *Political Psychology* 37, no. 2 (2016): 275–92; Bernard N. Grofman and Edward N. Muller, "The Strange Case of Relative Gratification and Potential for Political Violence: The V-Curve Hypothesis," *American Political Science Review* 67, no. 2 (1973): 514–39.

8   Jolanda Jetten et al., "A Social Identity Analysis of Responses to Economic Inequality," *Current Opinion in Psychology* 18 (2017): 1–5.

9   A critical analysis of the gig economy is provided by Alexandrea J. Ravenelle in "Sharing Economy Workers: Selling, Not Sharing," *Cambridge Journal of Regions, Economy and Society* 10, no. 2 (2017): 281–95.

10   Arundhati Roy, "Arundhati Roy: 'The Pandemic Is a Portal,'" *Financial Times*, April 3, 2020, https://www.ft.com/content/10d8f5e8-74eb-11ea-95fe-fcd27 4e920ca.

11   Intergovernmental Panel on Climate Change, *Special Report on Global Warming of 1.5° C*, United Nations, 2018, https://www.ipcc.ch/sr15/.

12   Gallup Polling, https://news.gallup.com/poll/1615/Environment.aspx.

13   Matthew J. Hornsey and Kelly S. Fielding, "Understanding (and Reducing) Inaction on Climate Change," *Social Issues and Policy Review* 14, no. 1 (2020): 3–35; Kimberly Doell et al., "Understanding the Effects of Partisan Identity on Climate Change," PsyArXiv, January 26, 2021, doi:10.31234/osf.io/5vems.

14   Matthew J. Hornsey, Emily A. Harris, and Kelly S. Fielding, "Relationships Among Conspiratorial Beliefs, Conservatism and Climate Scepticism Across Nations," *Nature Climate Change* 8, no. 7 (2018): 614–20.

15   Ibid.

16   Kimberly C. Doell et al., "Understanding the Effects of Partisan Identity on Climate Change," *Current Opinion in Behavioral Sciences* 42 (2021): 54–59.

17   Intergovernmental Panel on Climate Change, *Special Report on Global Warming.*

18   Frank White, *The Overview Effect: Space Exploration and Human Evolution* (Reston, VA: American Institute of Aeronautics and Astronautics, 2014); David B. Yaden et al., "The Overview Effect: Awe and Self-Transcendent Experience in Space Flight," *Psychology of Consciousness: Theory, Research, and Practice* 3, no. 1 (2016): 1.

19   Nancy R. Buchan et al., "Globalization and Human Cooperation," *Proceedings of the National Academy of Sciences* 106, no. 11 (2009): 4138–42; Nancy R. Buchan et al., "Global Social Identity and Global Cooperation," *Psychological Science* 22, no. 6 (2011): 821–28.

20   David Waldner and Ellen Lust, "Unwelcome Change: Coming to Terms with Democratic Backsliding," *Annual Review of Political Science* 21 (2018): 93–113; Nancy Bermeo, "On Democratic Backsliding," *Journal of Democracy* 27, no. 1 (2016): 5–19.

21   Sergei Guriev, Nikita Melnikov, and Ekaterina Zhuravskaya, "3G Internet and

Confidence in Government," *Quarterly Journal of Economics* (2021), https://doi
.org/10.1093/qje/qjaa040.

22 Kahn and Wiener, "Faustian Powers and Human Choices."
23 Bermeo, "On Democratic Backsliding."
24 Waldner and Lust, "Unwelcome Change."
25 Jennifer McCoy, Tahmina Rahman, and Murat Somer, "Polarization and the
    Global Crisis of Democracy: Common Patterns, Dynamics, and Pernicious
    Consequences for Democratic Polities," *American Behavioral Scientist* 62, no. 1
    (2018): 16–42.

INDEX

status, 142–45
Stephan, Maria, 199
stickers, 129–30, 141
Stone, Asako, 208
Stoughton, Seth, 56
strategic dissent, 212
stress, and group formation, 174–77,
    184–85
structural biases, 166–70, 173, 191,
    193–94, 195, 246, 268
Super Bowl (1984), 136
Swarthmore College, 64
Swiss identity, 48–49
symbols of social identities, 34, 102–3,
    123, 130–31, 144–45, 156–57, 244–45
system justification, 193–94

Tajfel, Henri, 15, 17
Taylor, Breonna, 155
teacher/learner electric shock experi-
    ments, 214–18, 220
teamwork, 187–91
Telzer, Eva, 161
Thatcher, Margaret, 235
threats
    evaluation of, 51–52, 56
    and group formation, 174–77
    leaders' response to, 246–48, 261, 274
    and social identities, 275
tokenism, 194
top-down attention orienting, 41
totalistic visions, 73–74
Tourish, Dennis, 72–73
toxic politics, 32–33
Toyota Prius, 141–42
transformational leadership, 238–39, 257
Tressel, Jim, 130
Truman, Harry, 238
Trump, Donald, 52, 89–90, 95, 102,
    106–8, 110–12, 115
trust
    and collaboration, 145–48
    and group formation, 12
    and leadership, 249–52
    and racial biases, 170–72
    and shared identities, 146, 249
    and social identities, 146–47
Truth and Reconciliation Commission,
    245
TWA Flight 741 hijacking, 174–76, 184–86

Twain, Mark, 263–64
Twelve Angry Men (film), 211–12
twenty-statements lists, 22–24
Twitter, 89, 95, 101–3, 105–9

Uber, 169
unconscious biases. *See* implicit biases
underdogs, 139
United States
    and charismatic leaders, 242
    and climate change, 269, 271
    and dissent, 203–5
    economic inequality in, 264–65, 267
    and individualism, 25
    presidential election of 2016, 102, 110
U.S. House of Representatives, 117–18
University of Alberta, 178–79
University of California, Berkeley, 248
University of Geneva, 88
University of Lancaster, 183
University of Minnesota, 61
University of Pennsylvania, 144
University of Queensland, 88
University of South Carolina, 56
University of Toronto, 26, 139, 179,
    216
University of Washington, 194
unjust treatment of groups, 12
unpleasant odors, 50–51
urban/rural norms, 27

vaccines, 88–89
Van Bavel, Jay J.
    and bystander effect, 177–82
    and collaboration, 145
    early college experiences, 3–4
    and group norms, 26–27
    and Stanley Milgram's electric shock
        experiments, 217
    and Ohio State University sports, 129
    rescue from choking by Dominic
        Packer, 4–6, 176
    and Stanford Prison Experiment, 259
    and study of identity, 7, 11–14, 157–61
    and twenty-statements lists, 24
van Linden, Sander, 91, 108
Van Vugt, Mark, 20
Vatcha, Naheed, 72–73
victim-blaming/shaming, 193
victim status, 262

ABOUT THE AUTHORS

Jay Van Bavel is an associate professor of psychology and neural science at New York University. From neurons to social networks, Jay's research investigates the psychology and neuroscience of implicit bias, group identity, team performance, decision-making, and public health. He lives in New York City with his family and pet hamster, Sunny, and once taught a class while trapped in an elevator with his kids.

Dominic J. Packer is a professor of psychology at Lehigh University. Dominic's research investigates how people's identities affect conformity and dissent, racism and ageism, solidarity, health, and leadership. He lives in eastern Pennsylvania with his family and their dog, Biscuit.

Jay and Dominic received their PhDs from the University of Toronto, where they bonded in a shared sub-basement office. This is their first book.